## *Front cover illustrations*

**Top left: figure 4.15**

Endoscopic view of right uncinate process and bulla ethmoidalis.

**Bottom left: figure 6.2**

Nasal inspiratory peak flowmeter in use.

**Top right: figure 6.5**

Acoustic rhinometry pre- and post allergen challenge.

**Middle right: figure 8.5**

Coronal CT scan showing mucosal thickening in the central nasal cavity
extending into the left infundibulum and ethmoids but with peripheral
pneumatisation (a black halo).

**Bottom right: figure 5.9**

Epithelial cells and enlarged goblet cells in nasal smear.

# Investigative Rhinology

## Glenis K Scadding MA, MD, FRCP

Consultant Physician in Allergy and Rhinology
Royal National Throat, Nose and Ear Hospital
Gray's Inn Road
London
UK

## Valerie J Lund MS, FRCS, FRCS (Ed.)

Professor in Rhinology
Institute of Laryngology and Otology
University College
London
UK

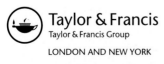
Taylor & Francis
Taylor & Francis Group

LONDON AND NEW YORK

A MARTIN DUNITZ BOOK

© 2004 Taylor & Francis, an imprint of the Taylor & Francis Group

First published in the United Kingdom in 2004
by Taylor & Francis, an imprint of the Taylor & Francis Group, 11 New Fetter Lane, London
EC4P 4EE

Tel.:      +44 (0) 20 7583 9855
Fax.:      +44 (0) 20 7842 2298
E-mail:   info@dunitz.co.uk
Website:  http://www.dunitz.co.uk

Although every effort has been made to ensure that all owners of copyright material have been acknowledged in this publication, we would be glad to acknowledge in subsequent reprints or editions any omissions brought to our attention.

Although every effort has been made to ensure that drug doses and other information are presented accurately in this publication, the ultimate responsibility rests with the prescribing physician. Neither the publishers nor the authors can be held responsible for errors or for any consequences arising from the use of information contained herein. For detailed prescribing information or instructions on the use of any product or procedure discussed herein, please consult the prescribing information or instructional material issued by the manufacturer.

A CIP record for this book is available from the British Library.

Library of Congress Cataloging-in-Publication Data

Data available on application

ISBN 1 84184 197 8

Distributed in North and South America by

Taylor & Francis
2000 NW Corporate Blvd
Boca Raton, FL 33431, USA

*Within Continental USA*
Tel.: 800 272 7737; Fax.: 800 374 3401
*Outside Continental USA*
Tel.: 561 994 0555; Fax.: 561 361 6018
E-mail: orders@crcpress.com

Distributed in the rest of the world by
Thomson Publishing Services
Cheriton House
North Way
Andover, Hampshire SP10 5BE, UK
Tel.: +44 (0)1264 332424
E-mail: salesorder.tandf@thomsonpublishingservices.co.uk

Composition by J&L Composition, Filey, North Yorkshire, UK

Printed and bound in Spain by Grafos S.A. Arte Sobre Papel

# Contents

# Preface

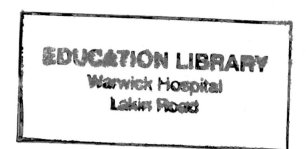
Which disorder affects approximately one billion people worldwide, reducing quality of life and working and learning ability, is also associated with serious sequelae such as asthma, sleep disorders, hearing problems and can be part of a systemic life-threatening vasculitis – yet is frequently dismissed, often not diagnosed at all, or misdiagnosed and frequently mistreated? Of course it is rhinitis – the Cinderella of respiratory tract disorders, largely ignored by chest physicians and left in the hands of primary care practitioners and ENT surgeons together with a few UK allergists.

Only a third of those with seasonal rhinitis, and 17% of those with perennial disease were satisfied with their treatment in a recent survey. Yet successful treatment of rhinitis can be very rewarding for both patient and practitioner. The starting point is accurate diagnosis – which is not always easy and is the reason for this volume. I was asked by Robert Peden at BACO in Cambridge over 4 years ago to consider writing a book on ENT and at first thought that I was too busy seeing patients, but then realised that passing on the methods which we use in clinics at RNTNE would benefit many more patients. The chapters cover history taking, examination of the patient (with a contribution from Valerie Lund on nasal endoscopy), and tests, including skin prick testing, radiology (again with help from Valerie), cytology, airways measurements, nasal challenge, smell tests, quality of life questionnaires and nitric oxide estimation. Advice is given on checking the lower airways, as suggested by the ARIA guidelines. Each chapter is extensively illustrated and an appendix contains useful documents such as history proformas, charts of predicted peak flow based on age and height and advice leaflets which can be removed and photocopied for use in the clinic. There is a list of suppliers of equipment such as Rhinoprobes, smell tests and acoustic rhinometers.

I hope that this volume will prove of use not only to ENT surgeons, but also to anyone who is faced with patients with difficult rhinitis.

Glenis Scadding, London 2004

# Preface

# 1

# The importance of rhinitis

Rhinitis which is defined clinically (Box 1.1), is the commonest immunological disorder in man. Recent figures suggest that it is a global problem affecting between 10 and 25% of individuals in different countries with increasing prevalence (Figure 1.1).

---

Box **1.1** Definition of rhinitis.

---

Rhinitis is an inflammatory disorder of the nasal mucosa characterized by two or more of the following symptoms:

rhinorrhoea (anterior and/or posterior)

blockage

itching/sneezing

---

Table **1.1** Rhinitis and asthma: quality of life.

| Health concept | Mean quality of life score (scale: 1–100) | |
|---|---|---|
| | Asthma ($n = 252$) | Rhinitis ($n = 111$) |
| Physical functioning | 80 | 89 |
| Social functioning | 84 | 73 |
| Role limitation (physical) | 66 | 61 |
| Role limitation (emotional) | 70 | 64 |
| Mental health | 66 | 65 |
| Energy/fatigue | 59 | 55 |
| Pain | 74 | 77 |
| Change in health (1 year) | 55 | 50 |
| General health perception | 57 | 62 |

1. Am J Respir Crit Care Med 1994; 149: 373
2. J Allergy Clin Immunol 1994; 94: 186
(Source: Bousquet et al. 1994a, b.)

Classically rhinitis has been described as a disease of no importance 'except to those who suffer from it'. In fact the symptoms have a marked effect upon quality of life similar to that experienced by sufferers with mild to moderate asthma and chronic back pain (Table 1.1). It is also a cause of missed attendance at both workplace and school (3–4% of the United States population), and of reduced productivity at both places (30–40%). The economic impact of rhinitis, or rhinosinusitis as it should be known since the sinus mucosa is nearly always involved, is significant: an estimated $5 billion per annum in the United States in 1996.

Rhinitis has significant comorbid associations related to its intimate connections between the nose, the sinuses, the middle ear and the lungs (Figure 1.2). These include asthma, sinusitis, pharyngitis, otitis media with effusion and sleep problems. Most is known about the rhinitis–asthma link (Box 1.2 and Figure 1.3).

The mechanisms of interaction between the nose and chest are not fully elucidated – certainly the ciliated pseudocolumnar respiratory epithelium is continuous from just inside the nose to the smaller bronchi and is likely to react in similar fashion all along its length. Other factors probably include nasal obstruction leading to

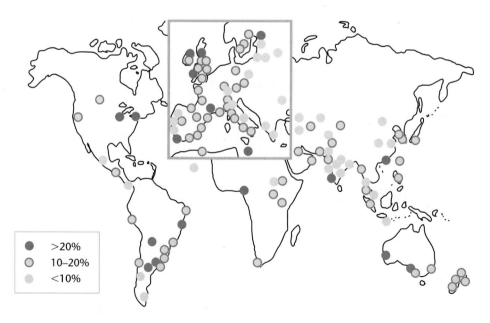

Figure **1.1**

The global prevalence of seasonal allergic rhinitis in 13–14-year olds: ISAAC. Data from the International Study of Asthma and Allergies in childhood. (Source: Strachan et al. 1997.)

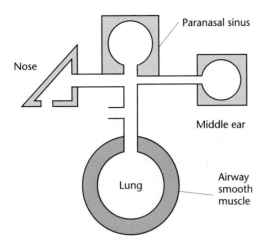

Paranasal sinus

Nose

Middle ear

Lung

Airway smooth muscle

Figure **1.2**

Nasal connections.

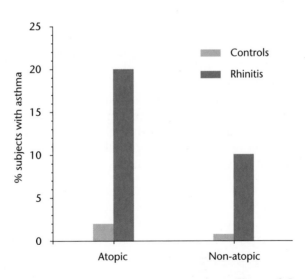

Figure **1.3**

Rhinitis, both atopic and non-atopic, is a risk factor for subsequent asthma. (Source: Leynaert et al. 1999.)

mouth breathing and loss of the normal filtration, warming and humidification of inspired air. The passage of postnasal secretions containing inflammatory or infectious mediators is unlikely to cause significant lower respiratory problems since it normally passes into the posterior pharynx and is swallowed rather than being inhaled. Naso-sino-bronchial reflexes exist; systemic connections

---

**Box 1.2** The rhinitis/asthma link.

---

Most asthma patients also suffer from rhinitis

Rhinitis, both allergic and non-allergic is a risk factor for the development of asthma (Figure 1.3)

Most asthma exacerbations start with upper respiratory tract inflammation – often viral, allergic or both

Rhinitis causes bronchial hyper-reactivity (BHR)

Treatment of rhinitis can decrease BHR and symptoms of asthma and reduce the need for emergency treatment

---

between the nose and lungs involving the production and release of eosinophil precursors bearing high affinity IL-5 (interleukin-5) receptors have been demonstrated. Nitric oxide, predominantly produced in the sinuses and upper respiratory tract, may also be relevant (see Chapter 7).

Thus, it is necessary to take rhinitis seriously to attempt as precise a diagnosis as possible, and to aim for successful treatment. The ARIA (Allergic Rhinitis and its Impact on Asthma, (Figure 1.4) guidelines provide a treatment plan for allergic rhinitis based on timing and severity (Figures 1.5 and 1.6).

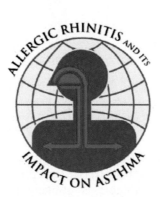

Figure **1.4**

---

The ARIA (Allergic Rhinitis and its Impact on Asthma) logo.

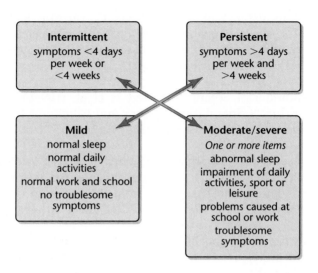

Figure **1.5**

Classification of allergic rhinitis

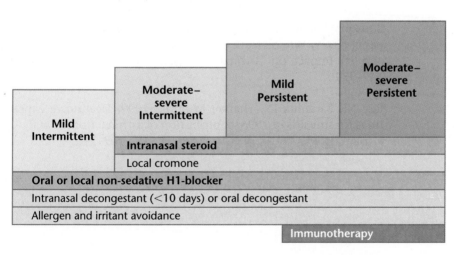

Figure **1.6**

The treatment plan for allergic rhinitis based on severity and duration according to the ARIA guidelines.

## References

Bousquet J, Bullinger M, Fayol C, Valentin B, Bustin B (1994a) Assessment of quality of life in patients with perennial allergic rhinitis with the French version of the SF-36 Health Status Questionnaire, *J Allergy Clin Immunol* **94(2pt1)**: 182–8.

Bousquet J, Khani J, Dhivert H et al. (1994b) Quality of life in asthma I. Internal consistency and validity of the SF-36 questionnaire, *Am J Resp Crit Care Med* **149(2Pt1)**: 371–5.

Leynaert B, Bousquet J, Neukirch C, Liard R, Neukirch F (1999) Perennial rhinitis: an independent risk factor for asthma in nonatopic subjects: results from the European Community Health Survey, *J Allergy Clin Immunol* **104(2Pt1)**: 301–4.

Strachan D, Sibbald B, Weiland S et al. (1997) Worldwide variations in prevalence of symptoms of allergic rhinoconjunctivitis in children: the International Study of Asthma and Allergies in Childhood (ISAAC), *Pediatr Allergy Immunol* **8**: 161–76.

## Further reading

Bousquet J, van Cauwenberge P, Khaltaev N and the ARIA workshop panel (2001) World Heath Organization Initiative: Allergic Rhinitis and its Impact on Asthma (ARIA), *J Allergy Clin Immunol* **108**: 147–334.

Ray NF, Baraniuk JN, Thamer M et al. (1999) Healthcare expenditures for sinusitis in 1996: contribution of asthma, rhinitis and other airway disorders, *J Allergy Clin Immunol* **103**: 409–14.

# 2
# Causes of rhinitis

The recent ARIA (Allergic Rhinitis and its Impact on Asthma) document has classified rhinitis and its differential diagnosis as shown in Boxes 2.1 and 2.2 (Bousquet et al. 2001). In practice, the simple division shown in Figure 2.1 is useful to bear in mind when investigating a patient. However, these divisions are not mutually

Box 2.1    Classification of rhinitis (ARIA).

**Infectious**
   viral
   bacterial
   other infective agents

**Allergic**
   intermittent
   persistent

**Occupational (allergic or non-allergic)**
   intermittent
   persistent

**Drug-induced**
   aspirin
   other medications

**Hormonal**

**Other causes**
   non-allergic rhinitis with eosinophilia syndrome
   irritants
   food
   emotional
   atrophic
   gastro-oesophageal reflux

**Idiopathic**

(Source: Bousquet et al. 2001.)

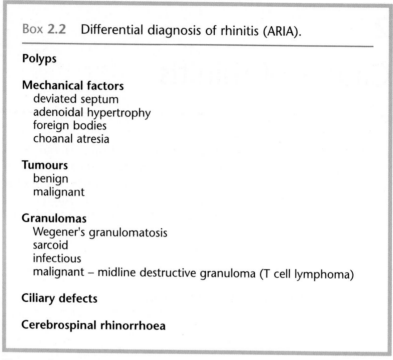

Box **2.2** Differential diagnosis of rhinitis (ARIA).

**Polyps**

**Mechanical factors**
 deviated septum
 adenoidal hypertrophy
 foreign bodies
 choanal atresia

**Tumours**
 benign
 malignant

**Granulomas**
 Wegener's granulomatosis
 sarcoid
 infectious
 malignant – midline destructive granuloma (T cell lymphoma)

**Ciliary defects**

**Cerebrospinal rhinorrhoea**

(Source: Bousquet et al. 2001.)

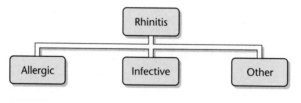

Figure **2.1**

This simple classification is useful when investigating a patient.

exclusive, for example allergic rhinitis may predispose to infection because of poor sinus or middle ear ventilation. Conversely, certain forms of infective rhinitis, such as that caused by the human immune deficiency virus (HIV) can lead to allergy since the gp120 subunit predisposes to Th-2 (T helper lymphocyte-2) cell formation.

# Allergic rhinitis

The pathophysiology of this disorder is complex and is detailed in Figure 2.2 which shows the early phase of the allergic response in the upper part and the late inflammatory phase in the lower part. It is now apparent that structural cells of the nose such as epithelial cells are also involved in this process (Figure 2.3). In fact, a simplified model (Figure 2.4) is useful for understanding the clinical symptomatology.

Allergic rhinitis was previously defined as seasonal or perennial, but now according to the World Health Organization ARIA guidelines

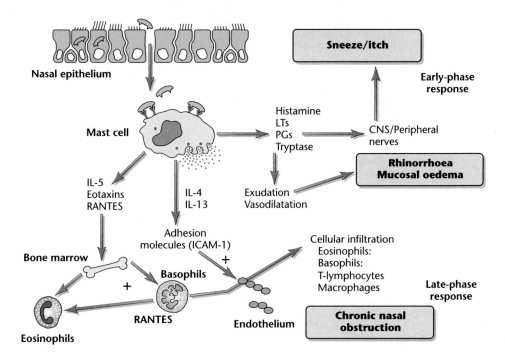

Figure **2.2**

The allergic cascade: the acute phase of allergic inflammation involves allergen contact with IgE (immunoglobulin E) molecules on the surface of mast cells which subsequently degranulate releasing mediators and cytokines. The major initial effects are sneezing, running and itching with blockage occurring after 15–20 minutes. Sometimes this is followed by a late phase allergic response: following mast cell degranulation there can occur a complex set of events involving further mediators, especially the leukotrienes, cytokines and chemokines which cause the influx of inflammatory cells, especially eosinophils. These cells in turn secrete further mediators and cytokines and can perpetuate the inflammatory response so that it persists for days or weeks. IL, interleukin; RANTES, Regulated on Activation Normal T cell Expressed and Secreted; LTs, Leukotrienes; PGs, Prostaglandins; CNS, central nervous system, ICAM, intercellular adhesion molecule.

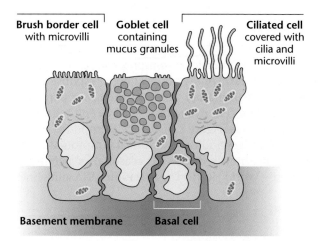

**Figure 2.3**

Other structural cells in the nasal epithelium such as epithelial cells, and nerves, are also intimately involved in the inflammatory process.

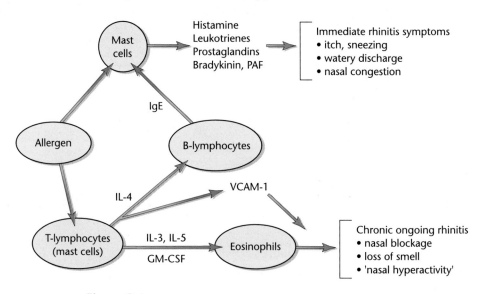

**Figure 2.4**

This simplified model of allergic disease is useful for understanding clinical symptomatology. In the early phase, the allergic response occurs soon after allergen contact with sneezing, itching and running being predominant features. However, when allergen contact is massive or chronic then the late phase predominates with symptoms being mainly of nasal blockage, any discharge passing posteriorly. The nasal mucosa is hyper-reactive and there is usually a diminution in olfaction. IL, interleukin; GM-CSF, granulocyte-macrophage colony-stimulating factor; VCAM, vascular cell adhesion molecule; PAF, platelet activating factor. Reproduced with permission of Professor Steven Durham.

'intermittent' and 'persistent' are the preferred terms since they are globally applicable (see Figure 1.5). Occupational rhinitis is increasingly being recognized, especially among healthcare professionals where latex particles on powder from latex gloves sensitizes those exposed, initially causing a rhinoconjunctivitis which can progress to asthma and anaphylaxis. The major causes of occupational rhinitis are shown in Table 2.1.

Table **2.1**    Most common causes of occupational rhinitis.

| Agents | HMW | LMW | Industry |
|---|---|---|---|
| Animal proteins | Dandruff, fur, urine, droppings | | Laboratory, breeding |
| Vegetable proteins | Grain/flour, latex | | Food processing, Bakers, Hospital workers |
| Enzymes (from animal and vegetable sources) | Papain, amylase, trypsin, cellulose etc. | | Manufacture, food processing, Detergents, Pharmaceuticals |
| Microbial agents | Antibiotics | | Manufacture |
| Chemicals | | Isocyanates Pinewood resins (colophony) | Plastic/paint Soldering (Electric trade)/ Glue |
| | | Acid anhydrides | Epoxy resins |

HMW, high molecular weight; LMW, low molecular weight substances.
(Source: British Society for Allergy and Clinical Immunology 2000.)

## Infective rhinitis

Most types of organism can infect the nasal mucosa (Box 2.3). Viral upper respiratory tract infections are common with each of us

Box **2.3**    Causative organisms of infectious rhinitis

Viruses

Bacteria

Mycobacteria

Fungi

Protozoa

Parasites

spending up to two years of life with common colds. These particularly affect pre-school children who suffer from 6–12 infections per year. By adolescence this decreases to 2–3 per year. Approximately

---

Box 2.4  **Bacteria which commonly infect the upper respiratory tract.**

---

*Haemophilus influenzae* (non-typeable)

*Streptococcus pneumoniae*

*Staphylococcus aureus*

*M. catarrhalis*

---

|  | **AFS** | **vs** | **EMR** |  |
|---|---|---|---|---|
|  | Ferguson, Laryngoscope 2000 | | | |
| • Mean age | 30.7 yrs | | • 48 yrs | p<0.001 |
| • Asthma | 41% | | • 93% | p<0.0001 |
| • Aspirin | 13% | | • 54% | p<0.0001 |
| • AR | 84% | | • 63% | p<0.004 |
| • Bilateral | 55% | | • 100% | p<0.0001 |
| • Mean IgE | 1941 mg/ml | | • 267 mg/dL | p<0.001 |
| • Polyps | 100% | | • 100% | p=NS |
| • M:F | 1.03 :1 | | • 1.26:1 | p=NS |
| • IgG | normal | | • IgG1 deficiency 50% | |
| • | fungal allergy in predisposed individuals | | • systemic immune dysregulation | |

Figure **2.5**

---

Allergic fungal sinusitis (AFS) is a clinically distinct entity from eosinophilic mucinous rhinosinusitis (EMR). *Key*: AR, Allergic Rhinitis.

80% of common colds in adults are caused by rhinoviruses of which there are around a hundred subtypes. Approximately 0.5–2% of viral upper respiratory tract infections progress to acute bacterial rhinosinusitis.

The bacteria which affect the upper respiratory tract are listed in Box 2.4. These tend to be carbohydrate coated and many of them have adverse effects upon mucociliary clearance. Rarer causes of rhinitis include mycobacterial diseases such as tuberculosis and leprosy. These are more common in the third world. *Klebsiella ozaenae* is found in association with atrophic rhinitis, but it is uncertain whether the organism is causative or a secondary pathogen.

The importance of fungi in nasal disease is hotly debated. The fact that fungi can be isolated from nasal secretions and are seen in association with activated eosinophils in patients with chronic rhinosinusitis has led to the suggestion that most cases, polypoid or otherwise, are fungal related. In contrast there is another view that fungi can be isolated from practically all noses, and there is a subgroup of patients with well defined allergic fungal rhino sinusitis which differs clinically from other rhinosinusitis patients with eosinophilic mucin (Figure 2.5).

# Drug-induced rhinitis

The overuse of alpha-agonists can cause rhinitis medicamentosa (Figure 2.6). Beta-blockers, and to a lesser extent other antihypertensive agents, can cause a chronically obstructed nose. Exogenous

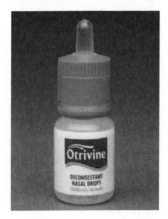

Figure **2.6**

Always ask about the use of over-the-counter medications, especially decongestant sprays which can cause obstruction (rhinitis medicamentosa).

hormones such as oestrogen in a contraceptive pill or hormone replacement therapy can also lead to rhinitis.

A subset of polyp patients shows exquisite sensitivity to aspirin and other COX-1 (cyclo-oxygenase-1) inhibitors. Concomitant asthma, usually intrinsic, i.e. skin prick test negative, is often found and may be difficult to treat. The new COX-2 inhibitors appear safe in the majority of aspirin-sensitive patients.

## Hormonal rhinitis

This is seen in pregnancy, and also at puberty and occasionally during the menstrual cycle. Hypothyroidism and acromegaly can also cause chronically blocked noses.

## Food-induced rhinitis

True IgE-mediated food allergy is an unusual cause of isolated rhinitis in adults, but rhinitis does occur as part of anaphylaxis. The oral allergy syndrome or birch-apple syndrome (see Appendix 1) occurs when a patient sensitized to tree pollens exhibits cross-reactivity to fresh fruits and vegetables.

Food intolerance can cause nasal symptoms. This can occur with chemicals such as dyes (E numbers) and preservatives (benzoates, sulphites and gallates) in non-allergic subjects. Aspirin-sensitive patients may also respond to these chemicals. Spicy foods, e.g. chilli cause rhinorrhoea probably because the capsaicin content stimulates sensory nerve fibres inducing peptide release. Recently, sensitivity to nickel in foods has been described as a cause of rhinitis.

## Atrophic rhinitis

This is characterized by atrophy of the mucosa and underlying bone. The nose is widely patent, crusted and odiferous. *Klebsiella ozaenae* is found, but may be a secondary problem.

Following extensive surgery secondary atrophy can occur.

## Autonomic rhinitis (*NENAR: non-eosinophilic, non-allergic rhinitis*)

Sympathetic nervous impulses dominate the nasal mucosa leading to the nasal cycle and a tonic vasoconstriction. Parasympathetic impulses cause rhinorrhoea and nasal congestion. Occasionally autonomic imbalance occurs leading to a blocked nose which pours with clear fluid, frequently at its worst first thing in the morning. The autonomic dysfunction is not confined to the nose, abnormalities are also noticeable in cardiac and postural reflexes.

## Non-allergic rhinitis with eosinophilia syndrome (*NARES*)

The extent of nasal smear eosinophilia necessary for this diagnosis (Figure 2.7) varies from 5–25% according to different authors. However, a recent study compared full thickness turbinate biopsies from patients with well-defined non-allergic rhinitis with allergic rhinitis turbinates and normal controls. The epithelium revealed mast cells and IgE positive cells present in both the intrinsic and allergic groups, but not in the normal controls (Figure 2.8). Nasal

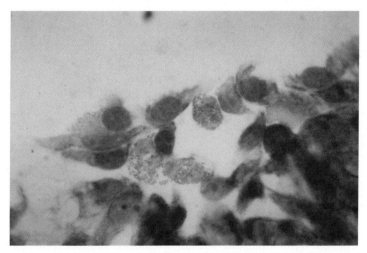

Figure **2.7**

Eosinophils seen in a nasal smear. The extent of nasal eosinophilia for the diagnosis of NARES varies from 5–25% according to different authors.

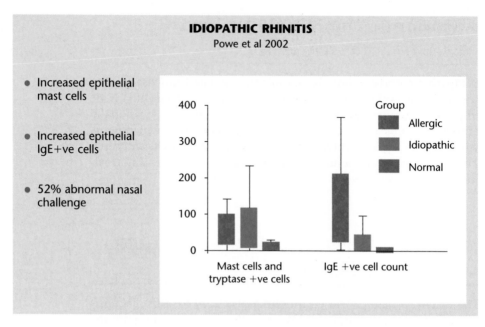

Figure **2.8**

Mast cells and eosinophils in inferior turbinates of patients with allergic rhinitis, idiopathic rhinitis and normal controls. (Source: data from Powe et al. 2002.)

challenges were abnormal in one half of the intrinsic rhinitis patients with definite positive responses in 20%. These results are in accord with others suggesting that local nasal allergy may occur and may be responsible for a proportion of NARES. This means that skin prick test negativity does not completely exclude allergic rhinitis.

## Other causes

Physical and chemical stimuli including dry air, pollutants and occupational irritants can cause rhinitis. Emotions such as stress and sexual arousal have a powerful effect on the nasal mucosa via the autonomic system. Gastro-oesophageal reflux can result in upper respiratory tract mucosal changes including rhinitis. This is more common in small children than in adults.

# Differential diagnosis of rhinitis

## Polyps

Nasal polyps can be classified in the same way as rhinitis (Figure 2.9). The most common form in the United Kingdom is the eosinophil-rich allergic type polyp (Figure 2.10), usually found in patients with negative skin prick tests. In contrast, in Thailand neutrophil-rich polyps predominate making up 80% of the total. Polyp associations are shown in Figure 2.11.

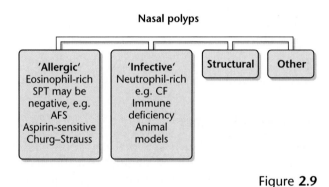

Figure **2.9**

Classification of nasal polyps. SPT, skin prick test; AFS, allergic fungal sinusitis; CF, cystic fibrosis.

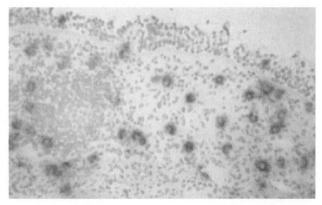

Figure **2.10**

Eosinophils in inferior turbinate from patient with aspirin-sensitive nasal polyposis. (Source: Varga et al. 1999.)

| NASAL POLYPS IN VARIOUS DISEASES | |
|---|---|
| Allergic rhinitis | 1.15% |
| Intrinsic (non-allergic) rhinitis | 5% |
| Atopic asthma | 5% |
| Intrinsic asthma | 13% |
| Cystic fibrosis | 6–10% (children) 50% (adults) |
| Aspirin intolerance | 30% |
| Churg-Strauss syndrome | 50% |

Figure **2.11**

Associations of nasal polyps.

## Mechanical factors

Mechanical factors such as septal deviation tend to cause nasal obstruction, often without significant associated symptoms, and are therefore not genuine rhinitis. Tumours, both benign and malignant, can affect any of the tissues in the nose or sinuses. In the UK, nasal tumours are rare ($< 1/100,000/$year). There are known predisposing factors, e.g. aniline dyes, wood dust especially hard woods with particles $< 5\,\mu$m in diameter and chrome pigments. There is usually a unilateral predominance not seen in inflammatory rhinitis.

## Granulomatous diseases

These diseases can present with a florid granulomatous rhinitis with crusting, contact bleeding and adhesions. Early diagnosis and treatment are important especially in the vasculitides, e.g. Wegener's granulomatosis (WG) and Churg–Strauss syndrome (CSS). In WG septal perforation or collapse (saddle nose) may occur, sometimes together with middle ear effusions, inner ear symptoms and/or laryngeal manifestations such as subglottic stenosis. In CSS there is an eosinophilic vasculitis (which can cause neurological complications) associated with nasal polyps and severe asthma. Sarcoidosis may present with nasal problems, usually with obstruction, crusting and contact bleeding again as a major feature.

## Ciliary defects

Primary ciliary dyskinesia (PCD) is found in approximately 1/10 000 individuals. Normal ciliary structure is shown in Figure 2.12. A variety of abnormalities have been found in PCD, including absence of inner or outer dynein arms or both, radial spoke and mitochondrial defects. Some PCD patients have structurally normal cilia but their arrangement is such that coordinated movement does not occur. Recently, however, a common defect – lack of iNOS (the inducible form of nitric oxide synthase) has been demonstrated in the nasal mucosa of all PCD individuals studied. There is a link between nitric oxide and ciliary movement which is as yet unexplained.

Secondary ciliary dyskinesia is common and can occur in response to infection, inflammation and pollution.

## Cerebrospinal rhinorrhoea

Cerebrospinal rhinorrhoea can follow a head injury, sometimes after many years, but is also found in those with no obvious preceding cause. The problem is almost always unilateral with clear watery rhinorrhoea which may be positional.  It may be associated with meningitis.

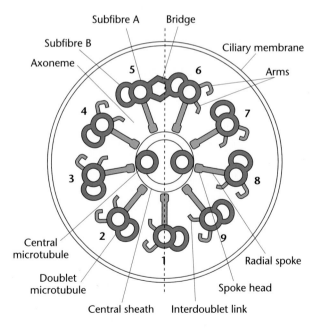

Figure **2.12**

Normal ciliary structure.

## References

Bousquet J, van Cauwenberge P, Khaltaev N and the ARIA workshop panel (2001) World Health Organization Initiative. Allergic Rhinitis and its Impact on Asthma (ARIA), *J Allergy Clin Immunol* **108**: 147–334.

British Society for Allergy and Clinical Immunology (2000). *Rhinitis: Management Guidelines.* Martin Dunitz: London.

Ferguson BJ Eosinophilic mucin rhinosinusitis: a distinct clinico-pathological entity. Laryngoscope. 2000 May; 110(5 Pt 1):799–813. PMID: 10807359 [PubMed – indexed for MEDLINE].

Powe DG, Huskisson RS, Carney AS et al. (2001) Evidence for an inflammatory pathology in idiopathic rhinitis, *Clin Exp Allergy* **31**: 864–72.

Scadding GK (1995) Rhinitis medicamentosa, *Clin Exp Allergy* **25**: 391–4.

Scadding GK (2001) Non-allergic rhinitis – diagnosis and management, *Curr Opin Allergy Clin Immun* **1**: 15–20.

Varga EM, Jacobson MR, Masuyama M et al. (1999) Inflammatory cell populations and cytokine mRNA expression in the nasal mucosa in aspirin sensitive rhinitis, *Eur Respir* **14**: 610–15.

# 3
# Making a diagnosis: history

To manage rhinitis effectively it is important to make as accurate a diagnosis of the condition as is possible. Most important is the fact that some potentially serious conditions can present with rhino-sinusitis. The major elements of diagnosis are shown in Box 3.1.

---

Box 3.1    Major elements of diagnosis.

History
Examination
Skin prick tests and/or RAST testing
Other tests

---

## History

An accurate detailed history is the most helpful guide to the nature of rhinitis. It can be time consuming, but a well-designed question-naire can shorten the consultation. The questionnaires used in our hospital are in Appendix 4 at the back of this book and are available for photocopying; however, you may wish to individualize them.

The first step is to note the major symptom – that which bothers the patient most. This is vital because rhinitis is a grey area and there is no clear division between symptomatic disease and normality. Patients may initially complain of one symptom such as nasal obstruction and then return with a different complaint, e.g. rhinor-rhoea or postnasal catarrh at a subsequent visit. The length of time for which the symptom has been present and when it occurs in the day, in the working week and in the year is important together with any factors which increase or decrease it. For example, in the United Kingdom seasonal rhinitis due to grass pollen usually begins in late May or early June and finishes at the end of July (Figure 3.1). House-dust mite sensitivity is a perennial problem, but tends to be experienced more during the autumn and winter months when people

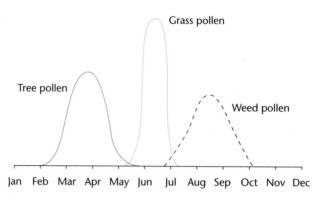

**Figure 3.1**

Allergen seasons in the UK. Spring hayfever is usually caused by tree pollens, the major ones being silver birch and plane trees which pollinate in April and May respectively. Grass pollens become troublesome in late May in the south east of England and cause symptoms until the end of July. After this, problems are usually due to weeds and nettle pollens as well as moulds and fungi. Housedust mites can cause symptoms all year round, but tend to be more problematical during the late autumn and winter months when houses are less well ventilated and more time is spent indoors.

spend more time indoors. It is frequently worse at night and in the early morning and may be exacerbated by household duties such as bed making and dusting. Work-related symptoms tend to abate during the weekend, but may not go away completely until there is a period of at least two weeks away from work.

Allergy to a pet in the home is not always obvious. Chronic obstruction may occur with symptoms of immediate allergy such as running, itching and sneezing only becoming apparent when the pet is re-contacted after a spell away. Bouts of itching and sneezing suggest an allergic process.

Non-nasal upper respiratory tract symptoms such as those involving hearing, ear ache, ear popping, tinnitus, sore throats (which can certainly occur following allergen challenge, but are usually more prevalent in infective disorders) and snoring may be volunteered by the patient. If snoring occurs then the patient should be asked about symptoms of sleep apnoea and daytime somnolence. The history from a partner may be useful here. The Epworth scale gives a useful guide to the severity of any sleep problem (Figure 3.2).

Since between a third and one half of rhinitics also have asthma, it is important to enquire about chest symptoms of shortness of breath, cough, wheeze and sputum production. Problems with mucociliary clearance or immune deficiency may also involve the lower, as well as the upper, respiratory tract. Such patients may have

# The Epworth Sleepiness Scale

Name: ................................................................    Date: ........................

Hospital Number: ..........................................................

How likely are you to doze off or fall asleep in the situations described in the box below, in contrast to just feeling tired?

This refers to your usual way of life in recent times.

Even if you haven't done some of these things recently, try to work out how they would have affected you.

Use the following scale to choose the most appropriate number for each situation:

    0: Would never doze

    1: Slight chance of dozing

    2: Moderate chance of dozing

    3: High chance of dozing

| Situation | Chance of dozing |
|---|---|
| • Sitting and reading | ❑ |
| • Watching television | ❑ |
| • Sitting, inactive in a public place (e.g. theatre/meeting) | ❑ |
| • Sitting, as a passenger in a car for an hour without a break | ❑ |
| • Lying down to rest in the afternoon when circumstances permit | ❑ |
| • Sitting and talking to someone | ❑ |
| • Sitting quietly after a lunch without alcohol | ❑ |
| • Driving a car, while stopped for a few minutes | ❑ |

Total Score: _____

Figure **3.2**

Epworth scale for sleep apnoea.

recurrent chest infections with production of thick greenish sputum. If the patient has bronchiectasis there is usually a quantity varying between a teaspoonful to an eggcupful produced on a daily basis.

Any other general symptoms may be relevant. For example, the patient with a vasculitis such as Wegener's granulomatosis or Churg–Strauss syndrome may complain of weight loss, tiredness, skin rashes or joint pains. Such symptoms may also be a manifestation of immune deficiency. Alternatively, patients who are allergic to tree pollens can have antibodies which cross-react with profilin present in many fresh fruits and vegetables. Thus the patient may have the birch-apple or oral allergy syndrome which manifests as itching or discomfort in the mouth on eating fresh fruit and vegetables, sometimes followed by throat discomfort and swelling and occasionally by gastric irritation (see Appendix 1).

Patients with the chronic fatigue syndrome (also known as myalgic encephalomyelitis or ME), may have an autonomic rhinitis, which appears to be part of their disorder. This is often accompanied by chronic tiredness, sleep problems and multiple other symptoms, sometimes including frank depression.

## Past history

This can include previous ENT problems such as tonsillitis or otitis media with effusion, possibly with operative intervention. This suggests that the basic rhinitic problem is longstanding. Allergy and immune deficiency are possible underlying factors. Allergic individuals may well have a previous history of atopic dermatitis in infancy or early onset of asthma or hayfever (Figure 3.3). A history of infection occurring at several sites such as urinary tract, sinuses and chest

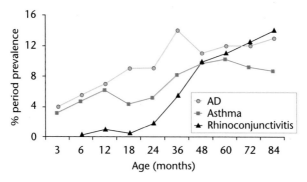

Figure **3.3**

The 'allergic march': the first manifestations of allergy are often food-related atopic dermatitis (AD) and/or gastrointestinal problems. Subsequently inhalant allergies usually become predominant with symptoms transferring to the respiratory tract.

suggests immuno-incompetence. The patient may have been previously infected with *Mycobacterium tuberculosis* or may be HIV positive.

## Family history

The importance of genetic factors in allergy is shown in Figure 3.4. However 15% of patients with allergic disease do not have a positive family history. It is also well known that nasal polyps run in families and having a father with nasal polyps gives a relative risk of 18 of polyps in the proband. The maternal influence is less strong with a relative risk of about 6. There may also be a family history suggestive of immune deficiency with other members having multiple infections. A history of infertility may suggest problems with mucociliary clearance.

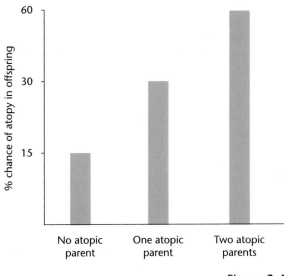

Figure **3.4**

Family history and allergy. The chances of being allergic are over 60% if both parents are atopic, 30% with one parent (more likely if this is the mother) and 15% with no family history of atopy.

## Social history

It is important to correlate skin prick test results with the patient's history and conversely the day-to-day life of the patient may suggest items to be included in the allergy work up. Factors predisposing to housedust mite in the environment are shown in Box 3.2. Recent building work in the home or a move to student accommodation are also possible causes of symptom exacerbation and hence referral to clinic.

---

Box 3.2 Factors associated with high HDM levels in homes.

---

Older homes (after 1940)

Older carpets

Condensation on bedroom/living room windows

Damp in any room

Mixed glazing

---

HDM, housedust mite. (Source: Simpson et al. 2002.)

Any contact with animals at home or at friends' houses, or at work should be sought. Patients often forget to mention that they have birds in the home. Exposure to animals in very early life and maternal exposure in late pregnancy appear to have protective aspects against the development of atopy (allergic reactivity). Other relevant factors include cigarette smoking or recent cessation (which appears to be associated with the onset of allergic symptoms). Exposure to multiple viruses at a nursery or day care unit may predispose small children to recurrent upper respiratory tract infections and otitis media.

## Occupational history

Occupational allergens fall into two groups: organic molecules and small inorganic molecules (see Table 2.1). Since occupational rhinitis usually precedes asthma it is an effective warning signal and every effort should therefore be made to diagnose and eliminate further allergen contact. This is because occupational asthma, once established, can become irreversible after a few months even after allergen exposure has ceased. Among healthcare workers latex sensitivity is becoming increasingly problematic and affects up to 18% of the healthcare workforce in some countries. Latex allergen is present on gloves that are powdered inside and therefore, unpowdered gloves are preferable or better still non-latex gloves made from vinyl. Latex allergy can be a cause of anaphylaxis and death – hence diagnosis is vital.

## Diet history

Many patients believe their rhinitis to be food related. Milk and other dairy products are commonly regarded as causing or exacerbating catarrh. As yet there is no definitive evidence for this. Milk allergy is very unusual in adults, but relatively common in small babies and infants where it can cause rhinitis, usually as part of a multisystem problem often involving atopic dermatitis, gastrointestinal symptoms including failure to thrive and possibly asthma. Eggs can give rise to similar symptoms in young children. In both cases the usual scenario is that the child usually loses the sensitivity at around the age of 3 years, but becomes sensitive to environmental inhalant allergens such as housedust mite and animal dander, and later on pollens. This is termed the 'allergic march' and the symptoms change from atopic dermatitis to asthma and rhinitis (see Figure 3.3).

In adults, food allergy is a very rare cause of rhinitis and, as in children, the rhinitis is usually accompanied by other symptoms such as oral allergy in the case of the birch-apple syndrome (see Appendix 1).

Patients with nasal polyps and with asthma who are aspirin-sensitive may also be sensitive to various additives and preservatives, the most common being alcohol. Approximately two thirds of the salicylate content of an aspirin tablet is found in certain foods, and a proportion of aspirin-sensitive patients (about 50% in our clinic) also have problems with these. The highest salicylate levels are found in herbs, spices, and preserves such as jams and jellies. Salicylate content of foods is variable, therefore, a well-defined list is not possible. However, we use the diet sheet shown in Appendix 2 as a guide for our patients.

## Treatment history

It is often helpful to find out which medications the patient has taken for his or her symptoms, how the medication was used and for how long. This way one often hears that topical nasal steroids were tried with a poor technique for a few days only before being dismissed as ineffective. Always ask about the use of nasal decongestants. Some patients are dependent on these and are suffering from rhinitis medicamentosa as a result. Although the literature suggests that effects occur within a few days of use, in fact it is almost always patients who have used topical decongestants regularly for a period of months who have the problems.

Other medications may be the underlying cause of a patient's symptoms – beta-blockers and to a lesser extent other hypertensive medications can cause nasal obstruction. The causative drugs are listed in Box 3.3.

---

**Box 3.3    Drugs causing symptoms of rhinitis.**

Beta-blockers

Other antihypertensives

Topical vasoconstrictors (if used regularly in the long term)

Oestrogen-containing preparations (oral contraceptives)

Hormone replacement therapy

Drugs causing hypothyroidism (chlorpromazine)

Aspirin and COX-1 non-steroidal anti-inflammatory drugs (only in sensitive individuals)

---

COX, cyclo-oxygenase.

Aspirin hypersensitivity can be latent. Always ask whether the patient can tolerate aspirin or non-steroidal anti-inflammatory drugs (NSAIDs) such as ibuprofen. If the reply is positive ask when these were last taken, since patients can develop sensitivity in middle age having previously tolerated such drugs. They may exhibit symptoms of rhinitis and/or asthma in response to aspirin-like foods or chemicals in food like E numbers and preservatives. Challenge with lysine aspirin can establish the diagnosis (see Chapter 5). If the response is negative ask for details of the symptoms which occur – gastrointestinal irritation is not necessarily associated with aspirin hypersensitivity in the respiratory tract.

## Reference

Simpson A, Simpson B, Custovic A, Cain Q, Craven M, Woodcock A (2002) Household characteristics and mite allergen levels in Manchester, UK, *Clin Exp Allergy* **32**: 1413–19.

# 4

# Examination

## External examination of the nose

Whilst taking a history it is simple to observe the patient for signs of breathlessness, hoarseness, nervousness, for coarse features of hypothyroidism or acromegaly, and to note their ability or otherwise to breathe through the nose. The face can give many clues including the allergic nasal crease and allergic salute (Figures 4.1 and 4.2). In allergic children, extra lines are seen under the eyes. Frequently there is also a high-arched palate in the allergic child whose face may well be pale, dry skinned and may show signs of atopic dermatitis (Figure 4.3).

The nose itself may be obviously deformed: there may be a deviation of the septum, a widening of the nasal bridge due to polyposis or other tumour (Figure 4.4), polyps protruding from the end of the nose (Figure 4.5) or discoloration such as lupus pernio in sarcoidosis. Collapse of the nasal bridge (Figure 4.6), formerly suggestive of syphilis, may now indicate previous septal surgery, Wegener's granulomatosis or midline lymphoma.

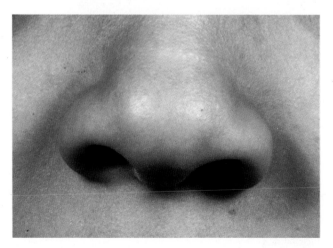

Figure **4.1**

Allergic crease.

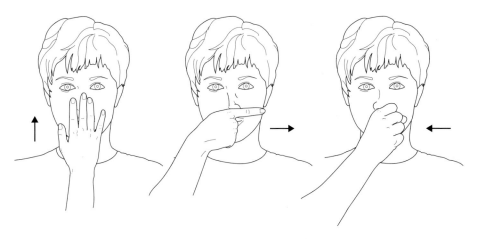

Figure **4.2**

Variations on the allergic salute.

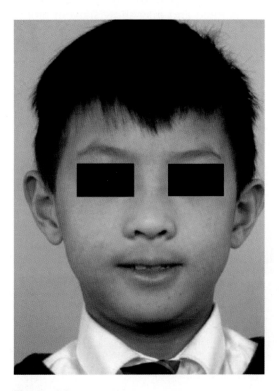

Figure **4.3**

Allergic facies: this child is an obligatory mouth breather with dry skin showing telangiectasia from chronic use of topical steroids for eczema.

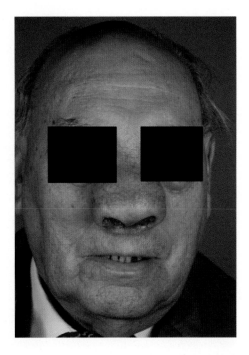

Figure **4.4**

Widening of the nasal bridge due to polyps.

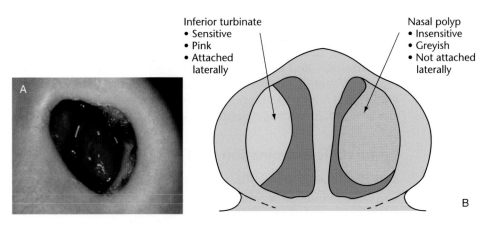

Inferior turbinate
• Sensitive
• Pink
• Attached
  laterally

Nasal polyp
• Insensitive
• Greyish
• Not attached
  laterally

Figure **4.5**

(A) Obvious polyps: these may conceal other pathology such as a tumour. (B) How to distinguish between hypertrophied inferior turbinates and nasal polyps (nose seen from below).

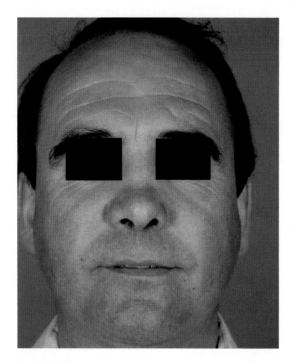

Figure **4.6**

Collapse of the nasal bridge due to Wegener's granulomatosis.

## Internal examination of the nose

Examination of the internal nose can be simply done in children and adults using an auriscope which gives a reasonable view of the inferior turbinates and the mucosa, lower airway secretions and lower septum. A slightly better view is afforded by the use of a head mirror and Thudichum's speculum. However, the best view of the nasal airway is obtained using nasendoscopes – rigid or flexible (Figure 4.7).

### Endoscopic examination of the nose

This is optimally done with a 30° 4 mm (or 2.7 mm) rigid endoscope. Sometimes it is necessary to prepare the nose with a local anaesthetic and decongestant such as Cophenylcaine forte (5% lignocaine (lidocaine) with 0.5% phenylephrine) or cocaine solution (5% or 10%) on cotton wool pledgets placed in the nose. However, it is always worth doing an initial examination to assess the mucosal appearances prior to shrinkage.

The endoscopic examination should be done in a systematic fashion. The first pass should be between the lower border of the

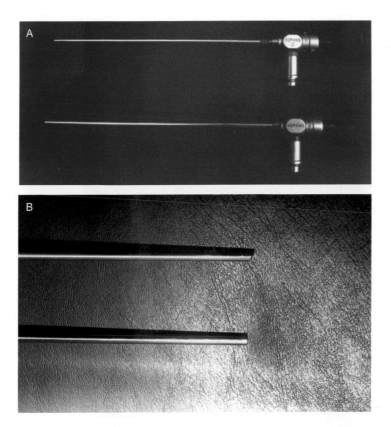

Figure **4.7**

(A) Hopkins rods used in nasendoscopy. (B) 0° and 30° nasendoscopes.

inferior turbinate and septum along the floor of the nose into the postnasal space (Figure 4.8). This is not possible in all patients and where specific examination of the nasopharynx is required, flexible nasendoscopy after decongestion should be performed. However, it is always important to check that the posterior choanae (Figure 4.9) are patent as unilateral choanal atresia can be sometimes present in young adults with unilateral nasal obstruction.

On the second pass, if the inferior turbinate has been surgically reduced and/or an inferior meatal antrostomy performed, the maxillary antrum may be viewed directly (Figure 4.10). Next, the region of the middle turbinate is carefully examined identifying the agger nasi region, at the junction of the middle turbinate anteriorly with the lateral wall of the nose (Figure 4.11). If this is pneumatized it may appear as a prominent bulge. The middle turbinate itself may be bulbous, indicating pneumatization (a concha bullosa), paradoxically bent or lateralized (Figure 4.12). In some patients it is possible to pass the endoscope between the middle turbinate and the septum to

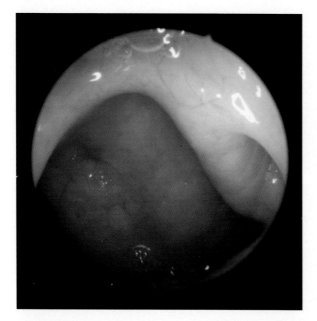

Figure **4.8**

Endoscopic view of postnasal space and left eustachian cushion.

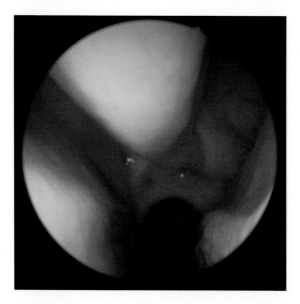

Figure **4.9**

Endoscopic view of posterior choanae and posterior end of middle turbinate.

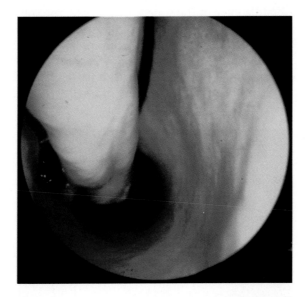

Figure **4.10**

Endoscopic view of right inferior meatal antrostomy.

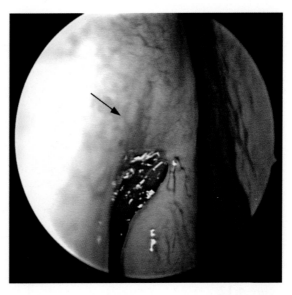

Figure **4.11**

Endoscopic view of right agger nasi region (arrowed).

obtain a view of the superior turbinate, the sphenoethmoidal recess and sometimes the ostium of the sphenoidal sinus (Figure 4.13). In some individuals a supreme turbinate is visible, a remnant of the ethmoturbinal system seen in lower animals. At this point it is worth looking up into the olfactory cleft particularly in patients complaining of problems with the sense of smell (Figure 4.14).

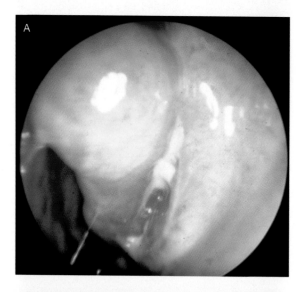

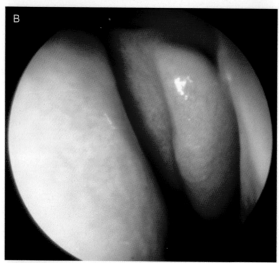

Figure **4.12**

(A) Endoscopic view of left concha bullosa. (B) Endoscopic view of left paradoxically bent middle turbinate.

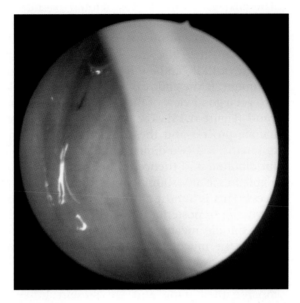

Figure **4.13**

Endoscopic view of left sphenoethmoidal recess and sphenoid ostium.

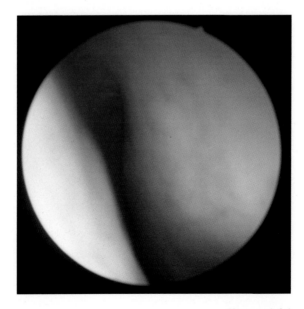

Figure **4.14**

Endoscopic view of left olfactory niche.

The next pass into the nose should examine the middle meatus. Sometimes is is possible to enter this directly between the anterior end of the middle turbinate and the lateral wall but more often it is easier to advance the endoscope along the inferior edge of the turbinate until it can be rolled up and laterally under its horizontal attachment. If the endoscope is now pulled back it is usually possible to get a good view of the uncinate process and bulla ethmoidalis behind (Figure 4.15). The gap between the posterior edge of the uncinate process and the anterior surface of the bulla, the hiatus semilunaris, is a two-dimensional space leading into the ethmoidal infundibulum and thence to the maxillary ostium. Sometimes it is possible to see an ostium lying anterior or posterior to the uncinate process. This is almost always an accessory ostium, lying either in the anterior or posterior fontanelle. The fontanelles are simply areas of the middle meatus where bone is not present but the gap is filled by the mucous membrane of the nose and maxillary sinus which may easily break down in the presence of acute infection. Accessory ostia are thought to be analogous to perforations in the tympanic membrane and are present in approximately 8% of normal individuals.

A conscious effort should be made to examine the nasal septum. A small pit about 1 cm from the front of the nose can be seen in

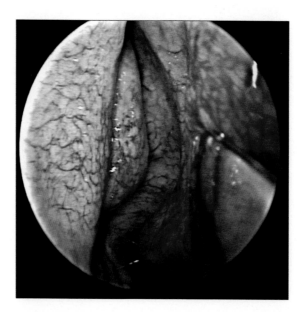

Figure **4.15**

Endoscopic view of right uncinate process and bulla ethmoidalis.

many individuals. This is the remnant of the vomeronasal organ, an accessory olfactory organ seen in lower mammals (Figure 4.16). The nasal septum may be deviated, in which case the inferior turbinate on the opposite wider side often undergoes compensatory hypertrophy. Spurs and dislocations of the septum from the maxillary crest may be observed and there may be holes in the septum as a result of previous trauma, surgery or disease (Figure 4.17).

An overall assessment of the mucosa should be made although colour and swelling per se are not specific to any particular disease. However, the presence of granular, friable mucosa would raise the suspicion of an underlying granulomatous process such as sarcoid or Wegener's particularly when associated with crusting and/or a perforation of the septum (Figure 4.18). The quality and quantity of the mucus should also be considered. Unilateral watery discharge which can be increased by bending the head forwards is strongly suggestive of a CSF (cerebrospinal fluid) leak. Thick, tenacious secretions may be associated with underlying mucociliary problems such as primary ciliary dyskinesia, and discoloration may indicate infection and/or a cellular infiltrate. Inspissated secretion described as resembling axle grease or peanut butter should immediately raise the suspicion of allergic fungal disease (Figure 4.19A,B). In addition to granulomatous conditions,

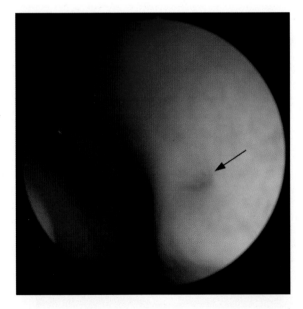

Figure **4.16**

Endoscopic view of right nasal septum showing pit of vomeronasal organ
(arrowed).

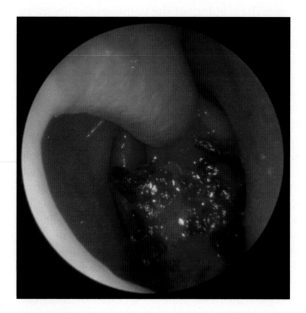

Figure **4.17**

Endoscopic view from left nasal cavity showing large septal perforation.

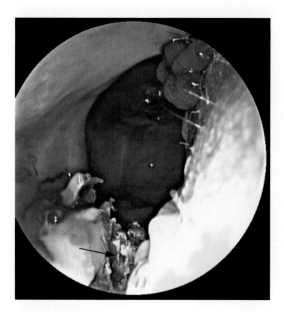

Figure **4.18**

Endoscopic photograph of lower part of nasal cavity showing crusting (arrowed).

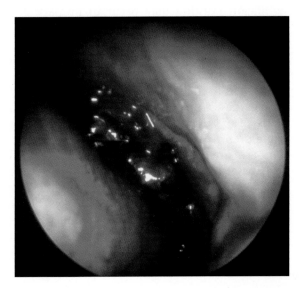

Figure **4.19A**

Endoscopic photograph showing typical appearances of secretions associated with allergic fungal rhinosinusitis.

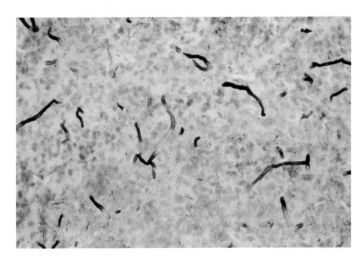

Figure **4.19B**

Grocott staining of secretion to demonstrate fungal hyphae.

significant crusting may occur in primary or secondary atrophic rhinitis.

Endoscopic examination will reveal the full range of pathology within the nasal cavity and give a strong indication of problems within the sinuses as they present in the areas of drainage on the lateral wall of the nose. Unilateral masses of any sort should always be regarded as potentially neoplastic and considered for formal biopsy. It is advisable to undertake imaging prior to this especially in children to establish the extent of the lesion and confirm that it is not a meningoencephalocele protruding through an anterior skull base dehiscence. Polypoid change is commonly seen in the nasal cavity most often affecting the lateral wall in the region of the middle meatus. It is almost always bilateral although often asymmetric in degree. The size of the polyps and other changes in the nose may be semi-quantified (Table 4.1) (Figures 4.20–4.22). Unilateral pathology should always raise the suspicion of neoplasia (Figure 4.23).

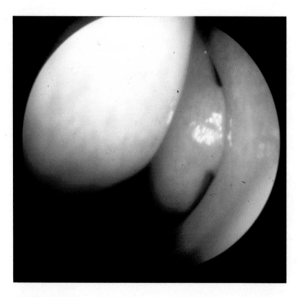

Figure **4.20**

Endoscopic photograph showing early polyp formation/mucosal apposition with localized area of oedema on left lateral wall.

Table 4.1  Endoscopic appearance score.

| Characteristic | Baseline | 3 months | 6 months | 1 year | 2 years |
|---|---|---|---|---|---|
| Polyp, left (0, 1, 2, 3) | | | | | |
| Polyp, right (0, 1, 2, 3) | | | | | |
| Oedema, left (0, 1, 2) | | | | | |
| Oedema, right (0, 1, 2) | | | | | |
| Discharge, left (0, 1, 2) | | | | | |
| Discharge, right (0, 1, 2) | | | | | |
| Scarring, left (0, 1, 2) | | | | | |
| Scarring, right (0, 1, 2) | | | | | |
| Crusting, left (0, 1, 2) | | | | | |
| Crusting, right (0, 1, 2) | | | | | |
| **Total points** | | | | | |

Polyps: 0, absence of polyps; 1, polyps confined to the middle meatus; 2, polyps beyond middle meatus but not completely blocking the nose; 3, polyps causing complete obstruction.

Oedema: 0, absent; 1, mild; 2, moderate/severe.

Disharge: 0, no discharge; 1, clear, thin discharge; 2, thick discoloured.

Scarring: 0, absent; 1, mild; 2, moderate/severe.

Crusting: 0, absent; 1, mild; 2, moderate/severe.

After Lund & Kennedy 1995

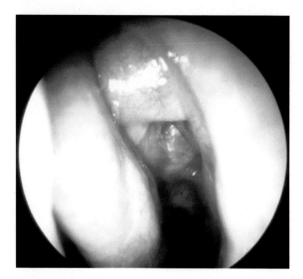

Figure **4.21**

Endoscopic photograph showing polyps within the middle meatus.

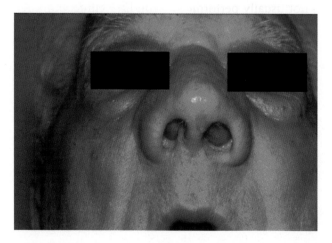

Figure **4.22**

Endoscopic photograph showing massive expansion of the nasal bridge and facial oedema in nasal polyposis.

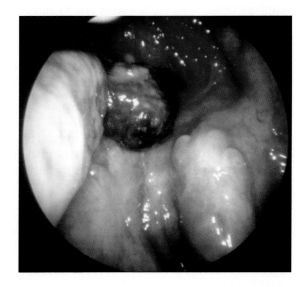

Figure **4.23**

Endoscopic view of surgical cavity with small recurrent malignant melanoma.

## Examination of the chest

The ARIA document (see Chapter 1) suggests that all patients with persistent rhinitis should be examined and tested for asthma. Chest examination is not usually performed in the ENT clinic, but a few simple observations should be made:

i    Is the patient breathless at rest, while talking or while walking?
ii   Is the respiratory rate high (>14/minute in an adult)?
iii  Is there any cyanosis or clubbing?

Routine examination of the chest includes inspection, palpation, percussion and auscultation.

### Inspection

With the patient sitting or standing and upper garments removed, look for abnormalities in chest shape. These include pigeon chest with a prominent sternum (pectus carinatum), often accompanied by indrawing of the lower ribs to form horizontal grooves (Harrison's sulci). This may occur following childhood asthma or upper respiratory tract obstruction. Pectus excavatum (funnel chest) is a localized depression of the lower end of the sternum or indeed its whole length. Thoracic kyphoscoliosis may occur, especially in older people or those with osteoporosis due to oral corticosteroids. Asymmetry of the chest may be seen in pulmonary fibrosis or collapse (Figure 4.24).

## Chest movements

It is helpful to watch the patient take a deep inspiration and expiration. In asthma the chest is usually hyperexpanded and lateral movement correspondingly reduced, instead the whole chest moves up and down during respiration. In normal healthy individuals, chest expansion of 5 cm or more occurs during inspiration (Figure 4.25).

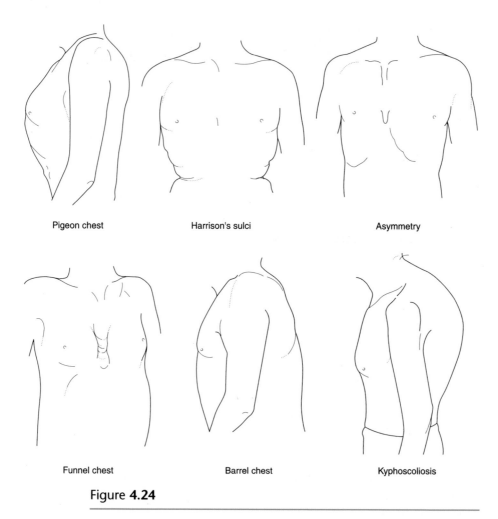

Pigeon chest          Harrison's sulci          Asymmetry

Funnel chest          Barrel chest          Kyphoscoliosis

### Figure **4.24**

Chest shapes.

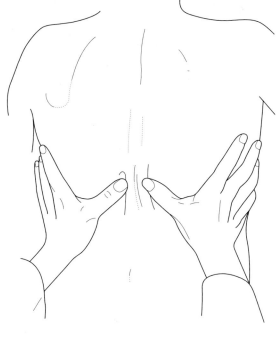

Figure **4.25**

Rough measurement of chest expansion with inspiration.

Palpation of the chest may reveal that the cardiac impulse is situated to the right of the sternum instead of the left leading to suspicion of Kartagener's syndrome.

Percussion is usually done both anteriorly and posteriorly comparing the two sides of the chest and the axilla. The normal note is resonant, this increases when air is trapped in the hyperexpanded asthmatic chest and decreases because of consolidation and over the liver. It becomes stony dull when an effusion is present. Auscultation is undertaken with the stethoscope, again comparing the two sides of the chest with the patient taking moderate breaths through an open mouth. Changes to note are variations in intensity or quality (bronchial breathing) and any added sounds such as rhonchi (wheezes) or rales (crackles) or even a pleural rub. The asthmatic lung can sound normal, wheezy or may be almost silent with very quiet breath sounds when airflow is greatly reduced. This last situation is associated with serious asthma requiring emergency treatment.

Some objective measurement of pulmonary function should also be made. This is discussed in Chapter 6.

Lund VJ, Kennedy DH (1995) Quantification for Staging Sinusitis. *Ann Otol Rhinol Laryngol Suppl* **167**: **104**: 17–21.

# 5

# Investigations

A few patients, for example those with seasonal allergic rhinitis, can be diagnosed on the basis of history and examination alone. Others require investigations to confirm or refute a putative diagnosis made on the basis of history and examination. The possible tests include:

- Allergy tests – skin prick or blood tests
- Other blood tests
- Other tests for allergy – nasal challenge and nasal smears
- Airway tests – static or dynamic
- Tests for the mucociliary apparatus
- Nitric oxide test
- Tests for cystic fibrosis
- Imaging
- Olfactory tests
- Test for CSF rhinorrhoea
- Nasal biopsy
- Microbiology
- Quality of life

Allergy tests and other blood tests are covered in this chapter. Airway tests are discussed in Chapter 6 and tests for the mucociliary apparatus, nitric oxide test and tests for cystic fibrosis will be found in Chapter 7. Chapter 8 covers imaging and the remainder of the tests are described in Chapter 9.

## Allergy tests

### Skin prick tests

▶ **RATIONALE.** An allergen introduced into the skin causes degranulation of IgE sensitized mast cells with mediator release and formation of a wheal and flare.

Skin prick tests are simple, cheap and safe provided food allergens are not used and no intradermal testing is undertaken. In Newcastle, there were three systemic reactions and no deaths over a period of 10 years when 32 000 skin prick tests were undertaken. Although systemic reactions are very rare, all skin prick tests must be undertaken with emergency equipment, including injectable epinephrine immediately available. Staff training in skin prick testing should include resuscitation training. It is our belief that all patients presenting to a rhinology clinic should undergo testing for allergy as a routine since chronic allergen exposure produces chronic nasal symptoms, the allergic nature of which may be missed unless the patient and physician are alerted to the possibility of allergy by positive skin prick test results.

## Method

A drop of a standardized allergen extract is placed on the volar aspect of the forearm and then introduced into the skin by pricking with a lancet (Figure 5.1). It is usual to test to a batch of allergens at the same time. A positive control (histamine) and a negative control (saline or diluent) should be included. A separate lancet is used for each test which is read as the mean wheal diameter at 15 minutes. Reactions greater than 2 mm in children under 5 years of age and 3 mm in adults are regarded as positive (Figure

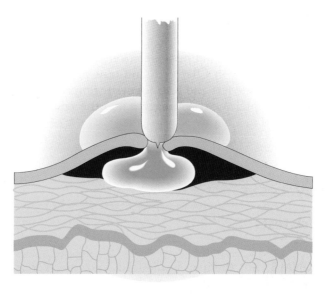

Figure **5.1**

Skin prick testing. The volar aspect of the forearm is used and the lancet is inserted at 90° to the skin surface through the drop of allergen.

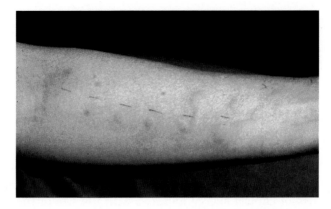

Figure **5.2**

Provided the negative control does not react and the positive gives a wheal the test is valid. Reactions greater than 3 mm are considered positive in adults, but may reflect sensitization and not clinical disease. Interpretation should be done in the light of the history.

5.2). Positive results should be at least 2 mm greater than the negative control. The wheal size relates to the amount of IgE, although the relationship is not linear. Tests in which the negative control gives a positive reaction are invalid, as are those in which there is no positive reaction to histamine. Under these circumstances RAST (radio-allergo-absorbent tests) should be employed.

A small battery of tests including a negative control, housedust mite, cat, dog, grass pollen and a positive control will diagnose the majority of rhinitis patients (Box 5.1). In the case of early hayfever, tree pollens may be included; a three-tree mix is available in the United Kingdom. However relevant plant allergens vary in different parts of the world and so local sensitivity patterns need to be checked. Other possible allergens include animals to which the patient has been exposed, moulds and occupational allergens such as latex.

---

Box **5.1**    Battery of skin prick tests which will diagnose over 90% of allergic rhinitics.

| | |
|---|---|
| Negative control (saline) | Cat |
| | Dog |
| Housedust mite | Positive control (histamine) |
| Grass pollen | |

### Exclusion

Skin prick tests should not be performed if the patient is on oral antihistaminics, has severe eczema, has had previous life-threatening anaphylaxis or has dermagraphism. Oral corticosteroids do not interfere except at very high dosage; dermal corticosteroids may reduce reactivity.

### Sensitivity and specificity

A positive skin prick test is not indicative of clinical allergy unless supported by the relevant history. Positive skin prick tests occur in 25–30% of adults, but only 10–15% develop symptoms. The risk of clinical allergy increases with the size of the skin reaction. Patients who have positive skin prick tests and no symptoms are sensitized: approximately half of these will go on to develop clinical allergic disease. Conversely, skin prick tests remain positive after the resolution of clinical allergy in some patients.

False negative reactions can also occur when allergy is localized. Recently, patients with intrinsic rhinitis were shown to have histological changes in inferior turbinates similar to those seen in allergy, and over 20% of these patients reacted positively on nasal allergen challenge (see Chapter 2).

Skin prick testing for food allergens is less reliable than inhalant allergens. False positive results are relatively common, false negative ones can also occur because commercial extracts are heat treated. If an unexpected negative result occurs to a commercial food extract, it may be worthwhile to undertake prick to prick testing with the fresh fruit, for example apple in the birch-apple syndrome.

### Intradermal tests

Intradermal tests are more sensitive, but less specific than skin prick tests (Figure 5.3). They are not recommended for the investigation of patients with nasal disease and have been largely abandoned in the United Kingdom since skin prick test extracts have become more potent and better characterized. They are occasionally used in the assessment of drug and venom allergy. In the United States, however, intradermal testing is common. It requires more technical skill and has a greater likelihood of producing systemic reactions.

## Blood tests for allergy

▶ **RATIONALE.** Stabilized allergen is incubated with the patient's serum, any specific IgE binds to the allergen and is identified by a second incubation with labelled anti-IgE.

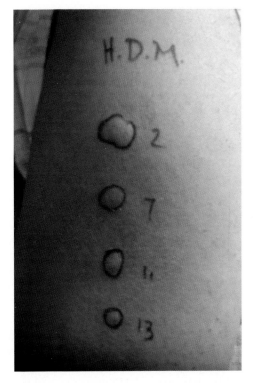

Figure **5.3**

Intradermal tests. These are more likely to cause a severe reaction and are less
specific than skin prick tests. They have no place in the ENT clinic.

## Total IgE

Total IgE is rarely helpful in uncomplicated rhinitis since 50% of
patients have IgE levels within the normal range. A more satis-
factory alternative is the Phadiatop test which involves the use
of several common allergens in a single test. It is reported as
either positive or negative and is more sensitive and specific in the
identification of atopy than is total IgE. However it does not give
individualized results for specific allergens and is unhelpful in
suggestions for allergen avoidance.

## Specific IgE

Specific IgE testing can be done with RAST or by fluorescent assays
and enzyme-linked immunosorbent assays (ELISA). RAST involves
incubating an allergen bound to a solid phase with the patient's
serum. IgE molecules bind to the allergen. After detailed washing
radiolabelled anti-IgE is added and the radioactivity is measured
after further washes (Figure 5.4). A recent improvement is the CAP

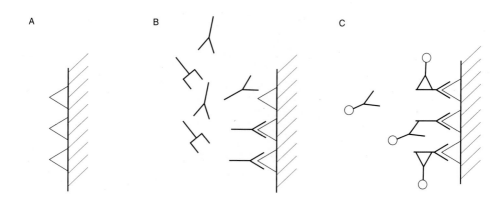

Figure 5.4

Principle of radio-allergo-absorbent tests (RAST). (A) Suspect allergen, e.g. egg bound to inert support. (B) This is incubated with serum from the patient. Anti-egg antibodies bind to the egg allergen. (C) After washing off unreacting antibodies labelled anti-IgE is added. After further washes the bound labelling is measured and compared to a standard curve.

RAST in which the allergen is coupled to a cellulose carrier and anti-IgE is enzyme-labelled with a fluorescent substrate acting as the developing agent. This system has a higher sensitivity and specificity than other RAST tests. The ELISA test is similar although the allergen is in the fluid phase and the IgE is enzyme-labelled. The substrate for the enzyme is added and the resulting colour change is detected photometrically. RAST tests are more expensive, delayed and no more sensitive or specific than skin prick tests. They should be used where the skin prick tests are contraindicated, or unavailable or difficult to interpret. There is usually good correlation between RAST and skin prick test results. RAST results show some relation to IgE levels. At very low levels of IgE ($< 20$ kU/l), it is unlikely that an individual RAST will be positive; at very high IgE levels, there may be false positives due to non-specific binding of IgE. RAST are often graded as 0–6 where 0 means no significant specific IgE, 1 is a borderline value and 2–6 indicate increasing levels of IgE. Box 5.2 shows a comparison between skin prick and RAST testing.

## CAST ELISA

The Cellular Antigen Stimulation Test involves sedimented leukocytes from patient blood which are simultaneously primed with the cytokine IL-3 (interleukin-3) and stimulated either with allergens or a suspect drug such as aspirin. Predominantly basophilic cells generate the allergic mediator sulphidoleukotriene LTC-4 and its metabolites LTD-4 and E4. These freshly synthesized leukotrienes are subsequently measured in an ELISA test.

> **Box 5.2    Comparison of SPT and RAST testing.**
>
> | SPT | RAST |
> |---|---|
> | immediate result | days to weeks |
> | cheap | expensive |
> | safe – inhalant only | very safe |
> | sensitive | slightly less sensitive |
> | affected by therapy | unaffected by therapy |
> | training for performance and interpretation | trained operator and interpreter required |

SPT, skin prick test; RAST, radio-allergo-absorbent test.

The difference in the leukotriene concentration in the sample stimulated by allergen (or drug) compared to the background sample (stimulated with buffer only) shows the releasability of the patient's basophils. A positive control is provided using a third blood sample from the patient stimulated with anti-IgE which should crosslink IgE molecules and lead to cell stimulation and leukotriene release. This should generate at least 300 pg/ml above the background level. Positive values for the test wells are thought to be greater than 200 pg/ml, the difference between the allergen stimulation and the background sample. As yet, the place of this test in allergy diagnosis is not established. There is some evidence to suggest that it correlates with skin prick test findings and with the results of allergen provocation. There is also a suggestion that it may be helpful in some food allergies and possibly in ASA (acetyl salicylic acid) sensitivity. However, in the latter case a negative result does not absolutely exclude an allergy or pseudo-allergy.

# Other blood tests

## Eosinophils in peripheral blood/eosinophil cationic protein

Isolated rhinitis rarely causes a blood eosinophilia. When associated with asthma, and especially when there is a systemic disorder such as aspirin sensitivity or Churg–Strauss syndrome (CSS), then peripheral blood eosinophil levels are elevated. It is also possible to measure one of the major proteins derived from eosinophils – the cationic protein or ECP. However, for the reasons mentioned above this is not particularly helpful in the diagnosis of isolated rhinitis.

## Full blood count

This basic investigation is needed in rhinitis of unknown cause or if recurrent infection or epistaxis is present. In children, the iron status should also be checked as iron deficiency is common in toddlers and can be associated with infections.

## Erythrocyte sedimentation rate (ESR)

This non-specific indicator of disease should be checked when a systemic cause of rhinitis is suspected. It can also be used to monitor therapy in such disorders.

## Serum immunoglobulins

Levels of IgG, IgA and IgM can be measured on a clotted blood sample by nephelometry in the routine laboratory. It is important to undertake this in patients with chronic or recurrent rhino-sinusitis as this can be the first manifestation of common variable immunodeficiency which appears in adult life. Hypogammaglobu-linaemia (IgG < 3 g/l) can be effectively treated by immunoglobulin replacement therapy.

## IgG subclasses

Four subclasses of IgG exist: IgG 1–4, with IgG 1 comprising about 60–70% of the total circulating IgG. Deficiencies in the remaining subclasses may be missed if only total IgG is measured. Since immune responses to particular organisms are often predominantly within a particular subclass, a deficiency of one may be associated with increased infections; however, some families lack complete subclasses without apparent problems. Most laboratories will under-take subclass analysis where the total IgG is under 11 g/l.

## Response to Pneumovax and tetanus toxoid

The dynamic response to immunization provides a better idea of immune status – this can be undertaken by your local immunolo-gist. The role of replacement therapy in subtle immune deficiencies is undecided.

## Thyroid function tests

Together with thyroid autoantibodies thyroid function should be tested where deficiency is clinically manifest and in unexplained obstructive rhinitis.

## Renal and hepatic function tests

Immune deficiency secondary to liver or kidney dysfunction occasionally presents as rhinosinusitis, therefore test these in unexplained cases.

## Anti-neutrophil cytoplasmic antibodies (ANCA)

The small vessel vasculitides – Wegener's granulomatosis (WG), microscopic polyangiitis (MPA) and CSS are all associated with circulating IgG ANCA versus autoantigens in neutrophil azurophilic granules.

ANCA (central or c-ANCA) against proteinase 3 (PR3) are strongly associated with WG and probably involved in the pathogenesis of this condition (Figure 5.5). However, early in the disease process the upper respiratory tract alone may be affected and ANCA are positive in around only 60% of patients. In these patients biopsy may be necessary. It is vital to biopsy an affected site, but even then results are often non-specific especially in the nose. Anti-myeloperoxidase (MPO) antibodies (peripheral or p-ANCA) occur in the other vasculitides, but can also be found in drug hypersensitivity reactions and diverse pulmonary disorders.

Recent analysis of tests for these conditions (which need to be accurate because of the use of cytotoxic therapy in treatment) suggests that both indirect immunofluorescence and antigen-specific tests need to be undertaken for both antigens, i.e. anti-PR3/c-ANCA plus anti-MPO/p-ANCA. This gives a sensitivity of 85.5% and a specificity of 98.6%.

ANCA titres do not accurately reflect disease, however, a four-fold rise in ANCA titre is thought to predict relapse. Simpler and quicker measures such as ESR, or depression of lymphocyte count may be more useful in monitoring disease activity.

## Angiotensin-converting enzyme

Angiotensin-converting enzyme (ACE) is a zinc metallopeptidase, which converts angiotensin 1 to angiotensin 11 and degrades bradykinin. It is elevated in plasma and in other biological fluids such as cerebrospinal fluid and broncho-alveolar lavage when local macrophages are activated. This occurs in granulomatous diseases

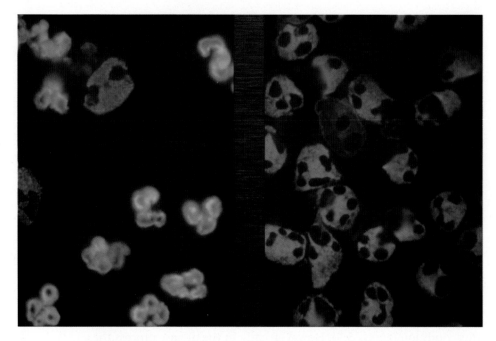

Figure 5.5

Indirect immunofluorescence showing anti-neutrophil cytoplasmic antibodies (ANCA). Wegener's granulomatosis is usually associated with central or c-ANCA (on the left), other small vessel vasculitides exhibit peripheral or p-ANCA (on the right). In fact, the positioning is a staining artefact and both types of antibody are directed against contents of neutrophil cytoplasmic granules: c-ANCA versus proteinase 3 and p-ANCA versus myeloperoxidase.

such as sarcoidosis and tuberculosis. Polymorphisms exist which cause large inter-individual variability and account for half the variance in plasma ACE level.

Other disease markers of sarcoidosis are a low lymphocyte count, CD4/8 lymphocyte ratio in induced sputum (which correlated with serum ACE in patients with uveitis) and depressed delayed hypersensitivity responses to recall antigens. Serum lysozyme can be used as a marker of disease activity. In suspected cases a chest radiograph may reveal asymptomatic bilateral hilar lymphadenopathy. Cysts in the bone may be seen on radiographs of hands and feet. Calcium studies should be undertaken to look for hypercalciuria.

# Other tests for allergy

## Vega testing

Vega testing employs electrodes attached to the body while the patient holds or is touched by allergen in a sealed container. It has been shown to be incapable of diagnosing common inhalant allergies.

## Kinesiology

The patient holds an allergen in a container with his or her arm outstretched. The examiner attempts to push down the arm, supposedly resistance is decreased when the patient is sensitive to the allergen being held. This method has never been verified.

## Nasal allergen challenge

This is the gold standard of allergy diagnosis, but is rarely necessary. Its place is where a positive history is accompanied by negative skin prick test.

▶ RATIONALE. Allergen is introduced into the nose and any reaction is measured and compared to placebo.

### Method
The relevant allergen needs to be obtained in a suitable form, i.e. not containing phenol or other irritants (Box 5.3). A placebo, preferably the diluent of the allergen, should always be employed initially. The allergen should be applied in gradually increasing concentrations with careful monitoring of both upper and lower respiratory tract symptoms. Both subjective (symptom scores, visual analogue scales, Figure 5.6), and objective (sneeze count, nasal inspiratory peak flow, rhinomanometry, acoustic rhinometry, spirometry or pulmonary peak flow) need to be employed. It is also possible to

---

Box 5.3    Methods of nasal allergen challenge.

Nasal spray – for general challenge purposes

Nasal drops – more useful in nasal polyposis

Pellet impregnated with allergen – most useful when a biopsy is required post challenge

**PATIENT'S RECORD**

NAME: _____ STUDY NO: _____

AGE: _____

SEX: _____

POTTED HISTORY: _____

----------------------------------------------------------------------------------------------------

DATE: _____

PRESENT RX: _____

LEVEL OF SYMPTOMS NOW: _____

Sneeze
├────────────────────────────────────────┤
0                                                              10
None                                                        Severe

Itch
├────────────────────────────────────────┤
0                                                              10
None                                                        Severe

Obstruction
├────────────────────────────────────────┤
0                                                              10
None                                                        Severe

Running
(Ant+Post)
├────────────────────────────────────────┤
0                                                              10
None                                                        Severe

Smear:

NIPF:

Rhinomanometry:

Washout with:                    ml of Na Cl              Vol. recovered =              Tubes No$^d$:

**Challenge with:**

10' NIPF:

Rhinometry:

Sneeze
├────────────────────────────────────────┤
0                                                              10
None                                                        Severe

Itch
├────────────────────────────────────────┤
0                                                              10
None                                                        Severe

Obstruction
├────────────────────────────────────────┤
0                                                              10
None                                                        Severe

Running
(Ant+Post)
├────────────────────────────────────────┤
0                                                              10
None                                                        Severe

Washout with:                                             Vol. recovered =              Tubes No$^d$:

Figure **5.6**

Visual analogue scale to assess subjective response to nasal challenge.

collect nasal secretions and measure mediators, cytokines or cells such as eosinophils.

Lysine aspirin, a truly soluble form of aspirin, can be used in this fashion as a test for aspirin sensitivity. Whereas with allergen the nasal reaction is immediate, occurring within 1–2 minutes and being maximal at around 15–20 minutes, with aspirin the reaction does not begin until about 45 minutes after nasal application and may persist for many hours (Box 5.4). Nasal aspirin challenge is considerably safer than oral or bronchial challenge with slightly lower sensitivity (Table 5.1). A negative nasal challenge should be followed on a later occasion by an oral one, starting with 30 mg of aspirin.

Nasal challenge testing is time consuming, difficult and requires extensive laboratory facilities. Resuscitation equipment and trained staff are also necessary.

Box 5.4    Comparison between nasal lysine aspirin and allergen challenge.

| **Allergen** | **Aspirin** |
|---|---|
| symptoms in minutes | symptoms after 45–60 minutes |
| airway changes in 20–30 minutes | airway changes similar |
| late response with high doses | late response common |
| increased asthma rare | increased asthma rare |

Table 5.1    Different challenges to assess aspirin sensitivity.

| History ± | Challenge | |
|---|---|---|
| | Sensitivity (%) | Specificity (%) |
| Oral | 77 | 93 |
| Bronchial | 77 | 93 |
| Nasal | 73 | 94 |

(Source: Nizankowska 2000.)

## Nasal smears

### Rationale
Nasal smears can be useful in determining the presence and type of inflammation present in the nose.

### Cost
Smears are simple and quick to take. The Rhinoprobe (Figure 5.7) is an excellent tool since its use is practically painless. Alternatively, a small bronchial brush can be used. The technique is to run the device from back to front of the nose along the inferior turbinate. This is undertaken three times on one side and the resulting material is spread onto a slide, fixed by a cryospray and then allowed to air dry. The process is repeated with a new probe in the other nostril. Staining is usually done with Wright–Giemsa. An alternative which is more complicated, but demonstrates eosinophils better, is Cresol-Red-O.

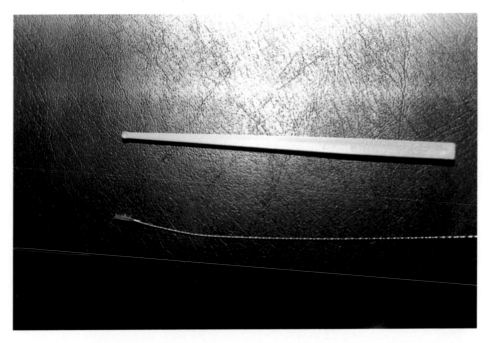

### Figure 5.7

Rhinoprobe (above) and bronchial brush. Both can be used to remove epithelial cells from the nose for cytology. However, the Rhinoprobe is more comfortable for the patient and gives an excellent result. It has to be imported from the United States, see Appendix.

The resulting slides need careful examination under the light microscope preferably by someone with cytological experience. This is time consuming since several hundred cells need to be counted on each slide.

## Reproducibility
Our studies suggest that the results obtained from the two sides of the nose can differ, possibly due to the nasal cycle limiting allergen ingress on one side. The cell content of smears varies with circumstances such as infection, irritants and allergen exposure, so that in asymptomatic periods smears may be normal.

## Interpretation
**Nasal eosinophilia**   Various authorities suggest figures of 5–25% for eosinophils in nasal smears as a nasal eosinophilia. This is seen in the allergic nose, but also in a condition called 'non-allergic rhinitis with eosinophilia' syndrome or NARES. First described by Jones in 1981 and often associated with bronchial hyper-reactivity, this is thought to be the forerunner of nasal polyposis and possibly aspirin sensitivity. However, since local nasal allergy appears to occur this could be a misnomer in some patients. The situation may need to be decided by allergen challenge. Our procedure is illustrated in Figure 5.8.

One reason for checking nasal smears is that eosinophil rich secretions suggest a response to topical nasal corticosteroids. However, it is often simpler to give a trial of drug therapy.

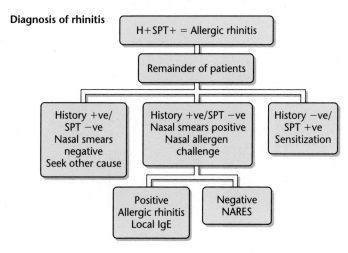

Figure **5.8**

Algorithm for the diagnosis of rhinitis. SPT, skin prick test; NARES, non-allergic rhinitis with eosinophilia.

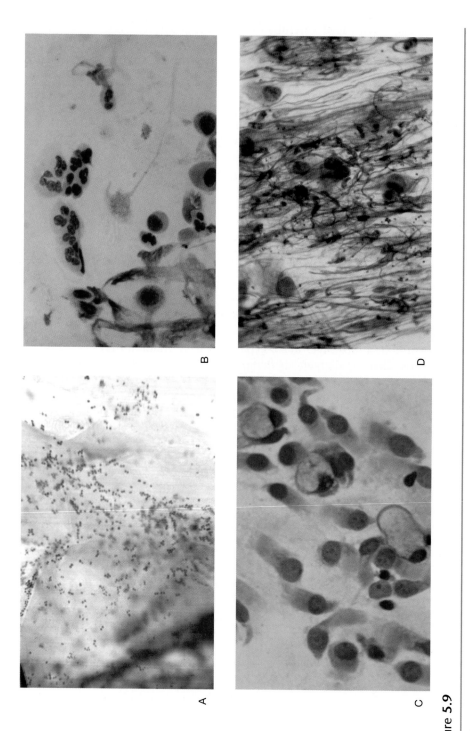

Figure 5.9

Nasal smears: (A) diplococii, (B) neutrophils, (C) epithelial cells and enlarged goblet cells (D) Ciliocytophoria – seen in viral infections.

## Other cells (Figure 5.9)

Neutrophils if plentiful are usually associated with bacterial infection, although some increase in neutrophils is seen during the allergic response. Bacteria themselves can frequently be seen in nasal smears, their shape and staining giving clues to their likely identity, for example Gram-positive diplococci are usually pneumococci. Shapiro (1985) has demonstrated that once the neutrophilia and bacteria are cleared by antibiotics the subsequent nasal smear may reveal eosinophilia.

Squamous cells may be noticeably abnormal in patients with work-related nasal symptoms such as ship-builders. Ciliocytophoria is seen in patients with viral infections. Fungi are not uncommon in nasal smears, although the significance of this is uncertain since fungi can be cultured from practically all noses.

From the foregoing, it can be concluded that nasal smears are unsuitable for routine investigation in every rhinitic patient; their use is necessarily restricted by the time and personnel available for cytological assessment. Their major place is in the work up of patients in whom rhinitis is difficult to classify, and in trials of treatment or allergen exposure or its treatment as a measure of response.

## References

Powe DG, Jagger C, Kleinjan A et al. (2003) 'Entopy': localized mucosal allergic disease in the absence of systemic responses for atopy, *Clin Exp Allergy* **33(10)**: 1374–9.

Nizankowska E, Bestyna-Hrypel A, Crniel C, Szczeklik A (2000) Oral and bronchial provocation tests with aspirin for diagnosis of aspirin – induced asthma, *Eur Respir J* **15(5)**: 863–9.

Milewski M, Mastalerz L, Nizankowska E, Szczeklik A (1998) Nasal provocation test with lysine-aspirin for diagnosis of aspirin-sensitive asthma, *J Allergy Clin Immunol* **101(5)**: 581–6.

Shapiro GG (1985) Role of allergy in sinusitis, *Pediatr Infect Dis* **4(6 Suppl)**, **5**: 55–69.

## Further Reading

Baudin B (2002) New aspects on angiotensin-converting enzyme: from gene to disease, *Clin Chem Lab Med* **40**: 256–65.

Brydon M (2000) *Skin Prick Testing.* Published by NADAAS, Norwich.

Choi HK, Liu S, Merkel PA, Colditz GA, Niles JL (2001) Diagnostic performance of antineutrophil cytoplasmic antibody tests for idiopathic vasculitides: meta-analysis with a focus on antimyeloperoxidase antibodies, *J Rheumatol* **28**: 1584–90.

Diamantopoulos II, Jones NS (2001) The investigation of nasal septal perforations and ulcers. *J Laryngol Otol* **115**: 541–4.

Scadding GK, Lund VJ, Darby YC, Navas-Romero J, Seymour N, Turner MW (1994) IgG subclasses in chronic rhinosinusitis, *Rhinology* **32**: 15–20.

Wiik A (2001) Anti-neutrophil cytoplasmic antibodies tests: which tests should be used in practice? *Intern Med* **40**: 466–70.

# 6
# Airway tests

## Nasal airway tests

It is possible to measure the nasal airway in a static or dynamic manner.

> ▶ **RATIONALE.** Although the airway is best appreciated endoscopically, measurements may be necessary if septal surgery is being considered or in the event of the symptom of nasal obstruction with an apparently normal airway. Objective airway measurements also improve the diagnostic accuracy of nasal allergen challenges and frequently form part of therapeutic trials.

### Spatula misting

When no other apparatus is available, the use of a cold spatula held under the nose whilst the mouth remains closed gives only a rough approximation of the nasal airway, although it does demonstrate whether nasal respiration is possible (Figure 6.1).

### Nasal inspiratory peak flow

This test involves the use of a peak flowmeter adapted with a nasal mask (Figure 6.2). It is relatively cheap, portable and can be used in much the same way as a pulmonary peak flowmeter to give information about the nasal airway with the patient in their normal environment or whilst taking medication. Not all patients can use the machine successfully. Adequate training is important; it is necessary to get a good seal with the facemask and to ensure that no oral inspiration takes place. It is sensible to give the patient a week's trial recording three values both in the morning and at night and to omit from trials any patient who cannot obtain values with a variation of < 15%.

Nasal inspiratory peak flow has several drawbacks. It is effort-dependent, and it is reduced by conditions such as alar collapse and

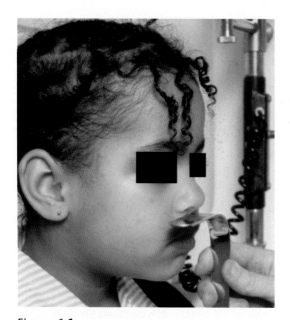

Figure **6.1**

Spatula misting – a rough guide to nasal patency.

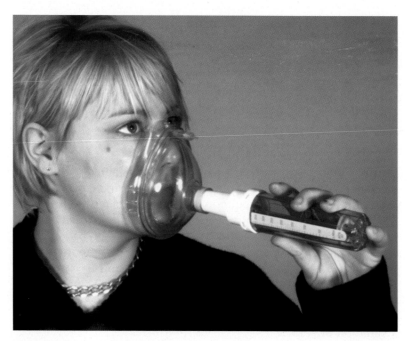

Figure **6.2**

Nasal inspiratory peak flowmeter in use.

lower respiratory tract conditions such as asthma and chronic obstructive pulmonary disease. There is no graph for expected values for age/height etc., but Box 6.1 shows a rough guide.

Box **6.1**    Nasal inspiratory peak flow.

| $< 50$ | – severe nasal obstruction |
| 50–80 | – moderate nasal obstruction |
| 80–120 | – mild nasal obstruction |
| $> 120$ | – no obstruction |

## Nasal expiratory peak flow

This test has been used, but can be uncomfortable for the patient since the eustachian tubes are inflated. It can also produce excessive mucus in the facemask.

## Rhinomanometry

Rhinomanometry measures nasal airway resistance by making quantitative measurements of nasal flow and pressure. This test is based on the principle that air flows through a tube only when there is a pressure differential across it. This differential is created by respiratory effort altering postnasal space pressure relative to that in the external atmosphere and resulting in air flow in and out of the nose. In 1984, the European Committee for Standardisation of Rhinomanometry selected the formula $R = \Delta P \div V$ at a fixed pressure of 150 pascals. This standardization allows comparison of results and the setting of normal ranges.

Rhinomanometry can be performed actively or passively, and by either anterior or posterior approaches. Active anterior rhinomanometry is the most commonly used, being most physiological. Pressure is recorded in one nostril by a catheter connected with adhesive tape, while flow is measured through the other open nostril. A transparent facemask is placed over the nose. This incorporates a pneumotachograph and is connected to an amplifier and recorder. The results are presented graphically as an 'S' shaped curve, with each nostril being measured five times. The mean value is used (Figure 6.3). The resistance at a fixed pressure of 150 pascals is expressed in 'SI' units.

Prior to testing, the patient should relax for 30 minutes in a steady temperature. The machine requires 30 minutes to warm up and needs regular calibration. Measurements are usually taken before and 10–15 minutes after nasal decongestion. This eliminates the effects of the nasal cycle and allows the reversibility of obstruction to be calculated.

Rhinomanometry is relatively time consuming and the reproducibility of results can vary by 20–25% within 15 minutes. It cannot be used when the nose is severely blocked or when there is a septal perforation. It does not assess the site of any obstruction.

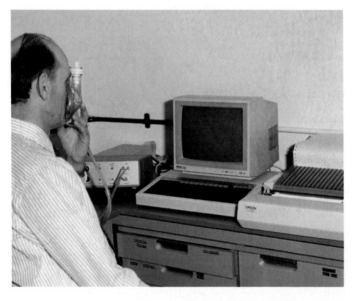

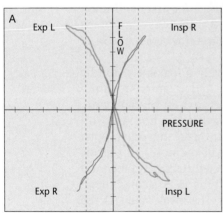
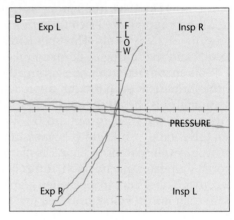

Figure **6.3**

Rhinomanometry tracings (A) Both nostrils patent. (B) Blocked left nostril.

In active posterior rhinomanometry, a catheter is inserted into the mouth with the lips closed around it in order to measure pharyngeal pressure. Flow through both cavities is measured simultaneously, although individual cavities can be assessed by plugging one at a time. The same transparent mask as for anterior rhinomanometry is used. This technique is less invasive and less likely to distort the nasal cavities. However, approximately one in four patients cannot relax the soft palate and some find it impossible not to suck on the tube. Results are again variable within a few minutes, usually between 15 and 20%. A day-to-day variation of 50% within an individual is possible.

## Acoustic rhinometry

Acoustic rhinometry employs an audible sound pulse (150–10 000 Hz), generated by an electronic click and propagated in a sound tube. It enters the nose and is reflected by local changes in acoustic impedance owing to changing cross-sectional area with distance (Figure 6.4). The reflected sound is picked up by a microphone,

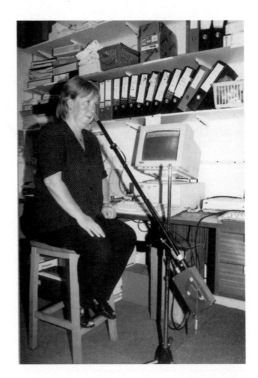

Figure **6.4**

Acoustic rhinometer in use.

passed to a computer and analysed, Fourier transformed and a read-out of cross sectional area versus distance from the tube obtained (Figure 6.5). The volume at different distances into the nose can be calculated.

Various nosepieces are available for attaching the sound tube to the nose. It is important that the nosepiece fits the nostril tightly without causing deformation. The acoustic tube should be held at the same angle on every occasion for each individual patient (a plumb line and protractor can be used to achieve this, alternative possibilities are a special headrest for the patient or a shadow tracing on the wall by a light which remains at one spot).

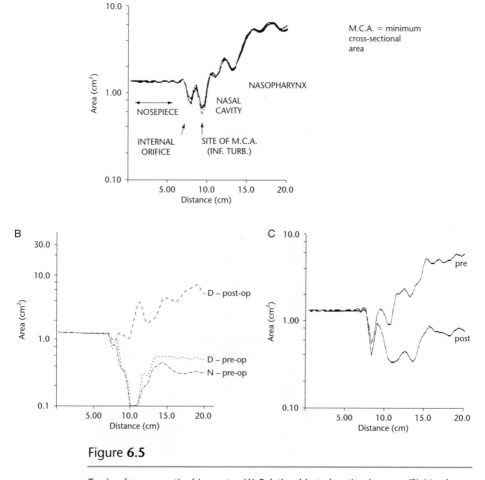

### Figure 6.5

Tracing from acoustic rhinometer (A) Relationship to location in nose. (B) Nasal polyposis – and pre- and post-operative traces. N = normal state, D = post-decongestant. (C) Pre- and post allergen challenge.

A train of five clicks is sent into the nose and the mean value used. It is usual to undertake this measurement, remove the tube from the nose, reposition it and repeat the measurement on at least one or sometimes two more occasions. During the measurement the patient can either hold their breath or exhale gently and slowly through an open mouth. A coefficient of variation is given for each run of five impulses, this is usually very low and the method itself achieves very reproducible results in the anterior part of the nose (around 7%), however, further back the variation is greater.

Again, it is usual to perform acoustic rhinometry both before and after decongestion.

The speed, ease and reproducibility of this technique make it very suitable for measurements during nasal airway challenges.

The positioning of a tube within the nose splints the anterior part of the nostril and may reduce alar collapse. In patients with anterior nasal obstruction, the use of acoustic rhinometry and nasal inspiratory peak flow tends to give contrasting results which may lead to this diagnosis.

Recently, the standardization committee on acoustic rhinometry has presented guidelines for quality control and optimal application of acoustic rhinometry. (Hilberg and Pedersen 2000)

i  A well-defined standard nose is used for testing and optimizing the equipment (data for a standard nose is given in the paper*).

ii  Procedures for evaluation of accuracy and repeatability of measurements in the standard nose are presented, and error limits are defined for the area-distance curve as a whole, for the minimum cross-sectional area and for the volume from 0 cm to 5 cm into the nose.

iii  Publication of results should include the volume 0–5 cm into the nose (volume from 2–5 cm for mucosal changes), the minimum cross-sectional area or preferably the two first minima and the distances to those areas.

iv  The operator should be trained, follow a standard operating procedure and the environmental conditions (temperature and noise) should be controlled.

v  Attention should be given to the nosepiece and the coupling between the equipment and the nose to obtain correct position and sufficient seal without disturbing the anatomy.

vi  The manufacturer should give information about the performance of the equipment, calibration procedures and maintenance, hygiene, environmental and safety standards.

## Rhinostereometry

Rhinostereometry involves microscopic examination of the nasal cavity with the patient's head held in a previously fitted frame. The

Table **6.1** Comparison of different nasal airway tests.

| | Spatula misting | NIPF | Rhinomanometry (anterior) | Rhinomanometry (posterior) | Acoustic rhinometry |
|---|---|---|---|---|---|
| Cost | Minimal | £100 | £6000 | £6000 | £6000 |
| Time | <1 minute | <5 minutes | 10 minutes + | 10 minutes + | <5 minutes |
| Difficulty | – | + | + + | + + + | + |
| Variability | Moderate | 10–15% | <20–25% | <20–25% | 5–10% |
| Standardization | – | – | Clement 1984 | Clement 1984 | Hilberg 2000 |
| Advantages | | Home use | | | Shows site of obstruction |
| Disadvantages | | | Need technical help | Need technical help | Need technical help |

NIPF, nasal inspiratory peak flow.

measurement is repeated after application of allergen, histamine or decongestant and the two-dimensional change in the inferior turbinate at the point of measurement is noted. This is a time consuming and difficult technique, and at present is practised in only one centre. It does not correlate with acoustic rhinometry.

## Manometric rhinometry

Boyle's law states that pressure times volume is constant for a given gas provided the temperature remains constant. This principle has been used to measure the total volume of the nasal airway plus sinuses. The idea seems excellent, however, as yet we have been unable to obtain reproducible results using the apparatus.

The different airway tests are compared in Table 6.1.

# Pulmonary function tests

A patient's own assessment of their asthma symptoms and severity is often poor, especially where air flow limitation is severe and long-standing. Objective assessment is necessary, preferably with a measure which is repeated after use of a bronchodilator to check reversibility of obstruction.

## Peak flow

The simplest test is peak flow in which the standing patient blows hard through a disposable filtered mouthpiece into a peak flow meter (Figure 6.6). Three attempts are made and the best is recorded. Charts of normative data relating peak flow to age and height are available.(see Appendix) If the result is not within the normal range the test can be repeated 15 minutes after administration of 50–100 µg of salbutamol or terbutaline to assess reversibility. A 20% increase suggests asthma. If there is a history of cough or wheeze on exercise then an exercise test such as running for 10–15 minutes followed by peak flow monitoring every 5 minutes will show a dip of over 20% if asthma is present.

Peak flowmeters are prescribable on the National Health Service in the United Kingdom, patients can be encouraged to record values at home in the morning and in the evening on a chart for a few weeks (Figure 6.7) and return with the results. A diurnal variation of over 20% suggests asthma.

These tests can be used in an attempt to diagnose the cause of cough, however, the ability to measure nitric oxide (NO) has decreased their use in our clinic, since elevated levels of expiratory

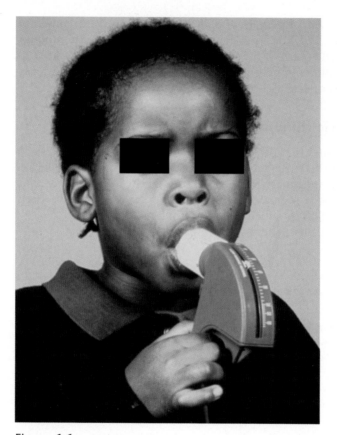

Figure **6.6**

Peak expiratory flowmeter in use.

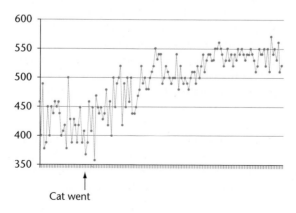

Figure **6.7**

Peak flow chart.

NO implies inflammation of some kind in the lower respiratory tract (see Chapter 7).

## Spirometry

The spirometer is a more expensive instrument which is not available for home use, but does give added information in the clinic. The patient is asked to blow maximally into a tube through a filtered disposable mouthpiece. This time the expiratory effort is continued until no more air can be expired. This is performed three times and the highest trace is used for measurements (Figure 6.8). The values noted are:

- FEV1 (forced expiratory volume in one second)
- FVC (forced vital capacity)
- Ratio of FEV1:FVC (this is over 75% in healthy adults, and over 85% in healthy children)

Normative data are available. The patterns of abnormal response include **obstruction** where FEV1 is low, FVC normal and the ratio reduced to below 75% and **restriction** where both FEV1 and FVC are low with a normal ratio. The former is characteristic of asthma and may be relieved by a beta-agonist, the latter of fibrosing or granulomatous lung conditions, such as sarcoidosis. An improvement in FEV1 of over 12% from baseline or an increase of 200 ml following inhalation of a short-acting bronchodilator is thought to indicate significant reversibility. However, some asthmatics

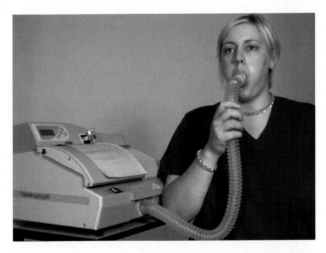

Figure **6.8**

Spirometer in use.

Table **6.2** Comparison of peak expiratory flow and spirometry in the assessment of possible asthma.

| | Setting | Advantages | Disadvantages |
|---|---|---|---|
| Spirometry | Clinic | Most reliable<br>Reproducible<br>Results seen in 15–30 minutes | Snapshot<br>Expense<br>Trained operator |
| Spirometry post-bronchodilator | Clinic | Best test<br>Gives best FEV results in less than 1 hour | Extra time |
| Peak flow | Clinic/home | Sensitive<br>Easy<br>Cheap | Less reliable than FEV<br>Patient compliance<br>Waiting period of ~4 weeks for home values |

FEV, forced expiratory volume.

only demonstrate this once inflammation in the airways has been reduced by oral glucocorticosteroids.

Peak expiratory flow and spirometry are compared in Table 6.2. Significant abnormality, when the patient has been encouraged to make a proper effort, should suggest referral to a chest physician.

## References

Clement PAR (1984) Committee report on standardization of rhino-manometry, *Rhinology* **22**: 151–4.

Fairbairn AS, Fletcher CM, Tinker CM, Wood CH (1962) A comparison of spirometric and peak expiratory flow measurements in men with and without chronic bronchitis, *Thorax* **17**: 168.

Gregg I, Nunn AJ (1973) *British Medical Journal* **3**: 282.

Hilberg O, Pedersen OF (2000) Acoustic rhinometry: recommendations for technical specifications and standard operating procedures, *Rhinology* **Suppl 16**: 3–17.

## Further reading

1995 Global strategy for asthma management and prevention. WHO/NHLBI workshop report, National Institute of Health, National Heart, Lung and Blood Institute Publication no. 95–3659.

Holmstrom M, Scadding GK, Lund VJ (1990) The assessment of nasal obstruction: a comparison between rhinomanometry and nasal inspiratory peak flow, *Rhinology* **28**: 191–3.

# 7

# Tests of the mucociliary apparatus, inflammation and cystic fibrosis

## Tests of mucociliary clearance

### Saccharin test

> ▶ **RATIONALE.** An innocuous substance with a sweet taste is placed in the anterior part of the nose, from where it will be moved backwards by mucociliary clearance. The time taken for it to reach the nasopharynx and posterior part of the tongue where it is tasted, is noted.

#### Method

The patient is asked to blow their nose. Under direct vision, using small forceps (Figure 7.1), a quarter tablet of saccharin is placed on the medial border of the inferior turbinate about 1 cm back from the anterior edge. The patient is asked to sit quietly without sneezing, sniffing, snorting, eating or drinking. They should swallow approximately once a minute and report as soon as any taste is experienced. The nature of the taste is not specified so that the patient can be asked about the quality of the sensation when reporting. A possible variation is to employ saccharin which has been dyed with Evans blue, so that this can be looked for in the nasopharynx.

Normal individuals have a saccharin clearance time of less than 20 minutes, longer times are seen in diseases where mucociliary clearance is abnormal such as primary ciliary dyskinesia (PCD) or cystic fibrosis, times may also be lengthened in chronic infective states such as chronic rhinosinusitis or in the acute viral cold. The prolonged test needs to be repeated on another occasion and if

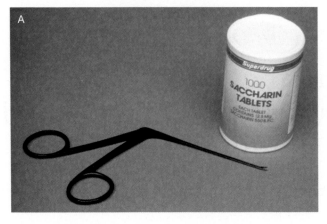

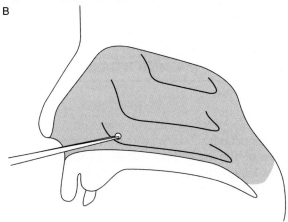

Figure **7.1**

(A) Crocodile forceps used for saccharin test. (B) Application of saccharin to inferior turbinate to assess mucociliary clearance.

persistently abnormal should suggest further investigation of mucociliary function.

## Isotope tests

It is also possible to employ a radiolabelled particle and monitor its progress using a scanner. However, this is expensive, involves radiation and is not available in most hospitals.

Mucociliary clearance can also be measured using identifiable probes during surgery. It must always be remembered that the application of local anaesthetic to the nose is likely to disrupt mucociliary clearance and give false results.

# Ciliary beat frequency

▶ **RATIONALE.** The beating frequency of cilia removed from the nose and held in Eagle's medium can be measured using a light microscope and photoelectric cell.

## Method

A sealed microscope cover-slide preparation is used for measurement of ciliary beat frequency. This is made by applying a thin border of grease using a 5 ml syringe and pipette tip around the edge of a cover slip to create a well. A Pasteur pipette is used to transfer the epithelium to the cover slip and a glass microscope slide is then gently placed over the cover slip, removing the air and sealing the preparation. The sealed preparation is then incubated at 37° C for 10 minutes to allow the sample to settle and equilibrate. The ciliary beat frequency is measured using a photometric technique (Dalmann and Rylander 1962). Slides are placed on an electronically controlled warm stage (Microtec, Oxford, UK) at 37° C and observed using Leitz Dialux 20 phase contrast microscope at magnification × 320. A strip of epithelium with beating cilia is chosen and the cilia are positioned to interrupt the passage of light through a small diaphragm, attached to a Leitz MPV microscope photometer. As the cilia beat they interrupt the passage of light from reaching the photometer and this is converted into an electronic signal which is then converted into beat frequency in Hertz (Hz) (Greenstone et al. 1984). For each sample, ciliary beat frequency is calculated as the mean of readings taken from 10 separated strips of randomly chosen strips of beating cilia. A record of the position of the epithelial strips is made from the same strip. Ciliary dyskinesia is defined as the absence of the normal coordinated pattern of ciliary beating (Figure 7.2) or a stiff appearance. The presence of ciliostasis, absence of ciliary beating, subjective length of the cilia and assessment of the epithelial integrity are recorded. When PCD is detected or there is a history suggestive of primary ciliary dyskinesia the sample is fixed in 2.5% cacodylate buffered glutaraldehyde (pH 7.2) in a round bottomed plastic tube and refrigerated for future electron microscopy.

This is time consuming and requires expensive equipment (Figure 7.3). It also needs a degree of technical expertise. However the method does lend itself to investigation of the effect of various substances upon cilia, albeit in vitro or removed from the nose after application of the test substance in vivo.

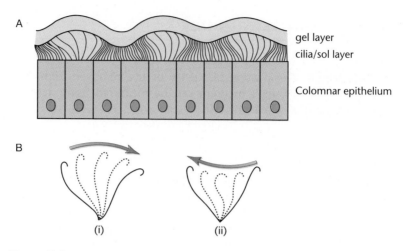

A

gel layer
cilia/sol layer

Colomnar epithelium

B

(i)            (ii)

Figure **7.2**

(A) Cilia beating in situ showing metachronistic pattern. (B) Normal ciliary motion (i) stiff forward stroke to move mucus, (ii) limp recovery stroke,

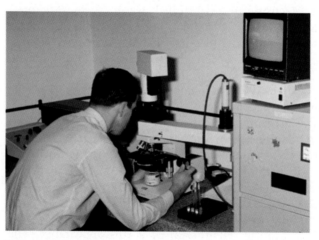

Figure **7.3**

Ciliary beat frequency analysis in progress.

Most cilia beat at 12–16 Hz when examined on a microscope stage and warmed to 37° C. The beat frequency is lower at room temperature. After four hours in culture, the cilia gradually lose their ability to beat and measurements are inaccurate.

# Electronmicroscopy of ciliary ultrastructure

When mucociliary clearance and ciliary beat frequency abnormalities are manifest, it is necessary to undertake electron microscopic examination of the cilia to see whether there are ultrastructural defects characteristic of primary ciliary dyskinesia (PCD).

Samples are processed a minimum of 24 hours after the sample has been taken for sample fixation. The supernatant glutaraldehyde is removed and after a change of cacodylate buffer (pH 7.2), the specimen is post fixed in 1% osmium tetroxide for 1 hour and then washed. Using a Pasteur pipette, a few drops of 2% agar (warmed to 42° C) are mixed with the specimen and centrifuged, before being solidified at 4° C. The agar embedded tissue is then processed for electron microscopy. Using a Lynx processor the tissue is dehydrated in a graded series of methanol: 70% for 15 minutes, 90% for 30 minutes and the 100% for 70 minutes. The tissue is then transferred to 100% propylene oxide for 60 minutes, to a mixture of 75% propylene oxide:25% araldite for 30 minutes, then to a mixture of 50% propylene oxide:50% araldite for 30 minutes and then to a mixture of 25% propylene oxide:75% araldite for a further 30 minutes. Prior to embedding in 100% araldite, excess agar is trimmed. Ultrathin sections (approximately 90 nn are cut using glass knives in a Reichert microtome. The thin sections are stained using lead citrate and uranyl acetate. This technique provides transverse and longitudinal sections of cilia with clear ultrastructural detail.

Transversely sectioned cilia are assessed at a magnification of × 30 000 (Figure 7.4). Sections are selected randomly from the

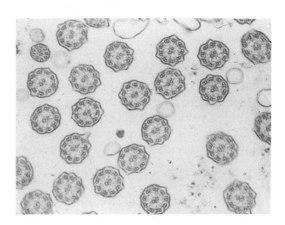

Figure **7.4**

Transverse section of cilia on electron microscopy.

epithelial strip. Microtubule abnormalities, compound cilia and dynein arms are identified and counted. Cross-sections of the samples are assessed for presence of both dynein arms, inner dynein arms only, outer dynein arms only, or for the absence of both dynein arms and for radial spoke associated defects.

## Measurement of ciliary orientation

Ciliary orientation is examined using an Improvision Image analysis system on an Apple Macintosh II-fx computer. The image captured on disk is retrieved on the computer screen. Ideally, for each sample, at least 10 good ciliary cross-sections from the same cell are required. On each image, a line is electronically drawn through the central pair of microtubules in each cross-section and the angle of each line is measured (vertical up = 0°, horizontal right = 90°, vertical down = 180°, Rayner et al. 1996).

This procedure is undertaken at a few specialized centres in the United Kingdom. It takes six weeks and is highly dependent upon technical expertise, and it is time consuming and expensive. Measurement of nitric oxide is an alternative method to largely exclude the diagnosis of PCD and may reduce the need for electron microscopy (vide infra).

## Hanging drop culture

Jorissen (2000 has suggested that examination of cilia removed directly from the nose may lead to inaccurate results since infection can not only reduce ciliary beating, but may also result in ultrastructural damage which can then be misattributed to primary problems. He advocates the use of hanging drop preparations in which the cilia are cultured for three weeks in a sterile environment. During this time, any secondarily damaged cilia regain their normal morphology. Electron microscopic examination is done after three weeks to detect those cilia which remain abnormal.

This very time consuming and expensive form of investigation is not at present undertaken anywhere in the United Kingdom.

## Nitric oxide

▶ RATIONALE. Measurements of nitric oxide in the lower respiratory tract, if elevated, represent some type of inflammation. Measurements from normal noses show a wide range of values and abnormal noses may give normal nitric oxide readings. However, the measurement may be useful in two ways: (a) very low values can indicate PCD or extreme nasal blockage, often due to grade III polyposis, and (b) elevated values suggest nasal inflammation and also ostiomeatal patency.

Nitric oxide, a free radical gas, is an important autocrine and paracrine messenger generated from arginine by a family of nitric oxide synthase (NOS) enzymes (Figure 7.5). Some of these enzymes are constitutive, the remainder are expressed by most cells involved in inflammation and are known as inducible NOS (iNOS). Nitric oxide has antiviral and antibacterial properties and plays a major role in innate immunity. Recently, nitric oxide has been found to stimulate ciliary mobility and to be absent or very low in primary ciliary dyskinesia.

Nitric oxide has been measured in the upper respiratory tract using the chemiluminescence principle, and tends to be elevated in inflammatory disorders such as allergic rhinitis, although levels are very variable. This is probably because constitutive nitric oxide production also occurs in the upper respiratory tract as demonstrated by Lundberg (2002), who punctured maxillary sinuses and found continuous production of nitric oxide (Figure 7.6). Presumably, it normally diffuses into the nose via the nose–sinus junction of the ostiomeatal complex (Figure 7.7) and this is reduced by obstruction from mucosal swelling or polyps.

## Nitric oxide measurement

In our laboratory nitric oxide levels (part per billion) are measured in nasal and exhaled air using an LR 2000 Logan Sinclair nitric oxide gas analyser according to the recommendation of Kharitonov et al. (1997). The subject sits relaxed and a probe is inserted into one

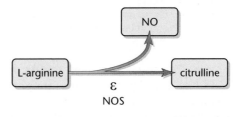

Figure **7.5**

Generation of nitric oxide (NO) from arginine. There are three varieties of nitric oxide synthase (NOS): neuronal and epithelial which are constitutive and an immune-related macrophage form which is inducible.

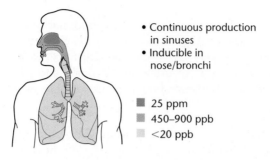

- Continuous production in sinuses
- Inducible in nose/bronchi

■ 25 ppm
■ 450–900 ppb
▫ <20 ppb

**Figure 7.6**

Nitric oxide in the respiratory tract. Very low levels are found in expired air (eNO), from the lungs unless there is some form of inflammation present in the lower respiratory tract. ppm, parts per million; ppb, parts per billion.

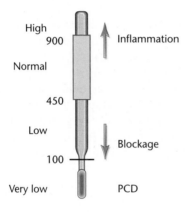

**Figure 7.7**

Nitric oxide levels in upper respiratory tract disorders. High nasal levels suggest inflammation and that the ostiomeatal complex (OMC) is probably patent; low levels suggest OMC blockage, or, if very low, grade III polyps or primary ciliary dyskinesia (PCD). Intermediate levels in the 'normal range' are those found in a population without nasal disease in our laboratory. Such levels in patients do not necessarily imply normality since they can be achieved by a combination of mucosal inflammation and sinus obstruction.

nostril. The subject is asked to take a full inspiration, and then to hold his or her breath to close the soft palate, while the nasal nitric oxide measurement is made. The nitric oxide value taken is that at the plateau that occurs after 30–60 seconds in most patients. Carbon dioxide is monitored in parallel to confirm that the soft palate is closed and that no contamination is occurring from the lower airways. Measurements are made in duplicate on both sides of the nasal cavity and the mean measurement is used.

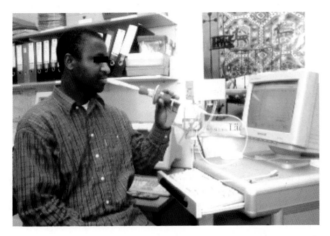

Figure **7.8**

Measurement of nitric oxide in expired air (eNO).

Pulmonary nitric oxide is measured with an oral probe while the subject exhales against a resistance sufficient to close the soft palate. Again, the plateau measurement occurring after 40–60 seconds is used (Figure 7.8). Measurements are made in duplicate.

# Tests for cystic fibrosis

▶ **RATIONALE.** Sinopulmonary infections may be a manifestation of cystic fibrosis. The presence of nasal polyps in small children, or of an affected sibling or parent or evidence of exocrine pancreatic insufficiency should prompt testing.

Cystic fibrosis remains a clinical diagnosis based on the presence of one or more characteristic phenotypic features (Box 7.1) plus laboratory evidence of elevated sweat chloride concentrations on two occasions, and/or laboratory evidence of two *CFTR* abnormalities or the in vivo demonstration of characteristic abnormalities in ion transport across the nasal epithelium.

Cystic fibrosis can vary considerably in the frequency and severity of clinical manifestations and complication. The diagnosis should not be discounted because a patient appears 'too healthy'. The subset of patients with pancreatic sufficiency is characterized by milder disease, better nutritional status and pulmonary function and a distinctly later age at diagnosis.

Box **7.1** Phenotypic features consistent with a diagnosis of cystic fibrosis (CF).

Chronic sinopulmonary disease manifested by:

(a) persistent colonization/infection with typical CF pathogens including *Staphylococcus aureus*, not-typeable *Haemophilus influenzae*, mucoid and non-mucoid *Pseudomonas aeruginosa* and *Burkholderia cepacia*
(b) chronic cough and sputum production
(c) persistent chest radiograph abnormalities (e.g. bronchiectasis, atelectasis, infiltrates, hyper-inflation)
(d) airway obstruction manifested by wheezing and air trapping
(e) nasal polyps; radiograph or CT abnormalities of the paranasal sinuses
(f) digital clubbing.

Gastrointestinal and nutritional abnormalities, including:

(a) intestinal: meconium ileus; distal intestinal obstruction syndrome; rectal prolapse
(b) pancreatic: pancreatic insufficiency; recurrent pancreatitis
(c) hepatic: chronic hepatic disease manifested by clinical or histologic evidence of focal biliary cirrhosis or multilobular cirrhosis
(d) nutritional: failure to thrive (protein-calorie malnutrition); hypoproteinaemia and oedema, complications secondary to fat-soluble vitamin deficiency.

Salt loss syndromes: acute salt depletion; chronic metabolic alkalosis.

Male urogenital abnormalities resulting in obstructive azoospermia.

## Sweat test

This remains the 'gold standard' for the confirmation or exclusion of the diagnosis of cystic fibrosis. Ideally, it should be carried out when the patient is stable, well hydrated, free of acute illness and not receiving mineralocorticoids. The guidelines of the National Committee for Clinical Laboratory Standards should be followed, with the test conducted by experienced personnel using standardized methodologies in facilities where adequate numbers of tests are performed to maintain laboratory proficiency and quality control. The only acceptable procedure is the quantitative pilocarpine iontophoresis sweat test. This can usually be carried out in the local paediatric department. A chloride concentration $>60$ mmol/l is consistent with the diagnosis of cystic fibrosis. Borderline concentrations occur in 4–5% of all sweat tests. The diagnosis should be made only if there is an elevated sweat chloride concentration on two separate occasions in a patient with one or more typical phenotypic features. In < 1% of cases the diagnosis of cystic fibrosis is established by other methods (nasal potential difference, genetic mutation analysis), such as in patients with borderline or normal electrolyte concentrations.

Other tests include DNA testing for the presence of mutations known to cause cystic fibrosis in each *CFTR* gene. To date more than 800 putative CF mutations have been described. In Caucasian populations the $\Delta^{508}$ is found in 68% of cystic fibrosis alleles. Both alleles need to be affected for cystic fibrosis, otherwise the patient is a heterozygote.

## Nasal transepithelial potential difference

Sinopulmonary epithelia, including that of the nose, regulate the composition of fluids that bathe airway surfaces by transport of ions such as sodium and chloride. This active transport generates a transepithelial electrical potential difference which can be measured and is raised in patients with cystic fibrosis compared to normal individuals. There is also a larger inhibition of potential difference after nasal perfusion with the sodium channel inhibitor amiloride. In cystic fibrosis, there is little or no change in potential difference when chloride free solution plus isoproterenol is used, reflecting an absence of CFTR-mediated chloride secretion. Basal potential difference can be measured at various sites throughout the nose using a catheter. For studying the response to perfusion with drugs, a double-barrelled setup is necessary. Again, the technique should be undertaken in a laboratory where these measurements are made frequently and need to be duplicated to be valid as a diagnostic adjunct.

The most commonly encountered errors in the diagnosis of cystic fibrosis are:

- Failure to consider the diagnosis because the patient is not Caucasian or looks too healthy or has normal pancreatic function
- Use of unacceptable sweat test methodology
- Misinterpretation of sweat test results because of inadequate sample, confusing values for sweat weight, osmolality and electrolyte concentration; failure to repeat positive and borderline results and failure to repeat a negative sweat test in a patient with a highly suggestive clinical picture
- Failure to consider the diagnosis in a patient who does not follow the usual or expected clinical course.

In considering atypical cases, computerized tomography (CT) may be helpful in that normal radiographic and CT findings provide strong evidence against a diagnosis of cystic fibrosis. Homogeneous opacification of the paranasal sinuses (especially maxillary), is a constant finding in almost all patients past infancy. Bilateral medial displacement of the lateral nasal wall and uncinate process demineralization are particularly suggestive of cystic fibrosis.

## References

Greenstone M, Cole PJ (1984) Primary ciliary dyskinesia, *Arch Dis Child* **59(8)**: 704–6.

Jorissen M, Willems T, Van der Schueren B, Verbeken E (2000) Secondary ciliary dyskinesia is absent after ciliogenesis in culture, *Acta Otorhinolaryngol Belg* **54(3)**: 333–42

Kharitonov S, Alving K, Barnes PJ (1997) Exhaled and nasal nitric oxide measurements: recommendations. The European Respiratory Society Task Force, *Eur Respir J* **10(7)**: 1683–93.

Lundberg JO, Palm J, Alving K (2002) Nitric oxide but not carbon monoxide is continuously released in the human nasal airways, *Eur Respir J* **20(1)**: 100–3

Rayner CF, Rutman A, Dewar A et al. (1996) Ciliary disorientation alone as a cause of primary ciliary dyskinesia syndrome, *Am J Respir Crit Care Med* **153(3)**: 1123–9.

Stanley P, MacWilliam L, Greenstone M, Mackay I, Cole P (1984) Efficacy of a saccharin test for screening to detect abnormal mucociliary clearance, *Br J Dis Chest* **78(1)**: 62–5.

Tornberg DC, Marteus H, Schedin U et al. (2002) Nasal and oral contribution to inhaled and exhaled nitric oxide: a study in tracheotomized patients, *Eur Respir J* **19(5)**: 859–64.

Wodehouse T, Kharitonov SA, Mackay IS et al. (2003) Nasal nitric oxide measurements for the screening of primary ciliary dyskinesia, *Eur Respir J* **21(1)**: 43–7.

## Further reading

Rosenstein BJ (2000) Diagnostic methods In: Hobson ME , Geddes DM, eds, Cystic Fibrosis. Arnold

# 8

# Imaging

Plain radiographs have been superseded in virtually all cases by computerized tomography for the demonstration of inflammatory and infective conditions. For more serious pathology such as tumours, magnetic resonance imaging (MRI) is often added, together with magnetic resonance angiography (MRA), positron emission tomography (PET) scanning and ultrasound in selected cases.

Computerized tomography (CT) is the 'gold standard' for demonstrating extent of disease and fine detailed anatomy, both prerequisites if surgery is to be undertaken. However, scanning is usually reserved until such surgery is contemplated, usually only after an adequate trial of medical therapy. Exceptions to this are patients with unilateral disease or where there is suspicion of malignancy. A variety of protocols minimizing radiation dose to the lens whilst providing high quality images are available, of which an example is shown in Table 8.1.

When evaluating a CT scan estimation of disease extent is possible using a number of staging and scoring systems, one of the more popular of which is the Lund–Mackay system (Table 8.2). The anatomical features which should be evaluated on the scan are shown in Box 8.1.

Table **8.1** Example of protocol for computerized tomography in chronic rhinosinusitis.*

| | |
|---|---|
| Plane | Direct coronal |
| Slice thickness | 5 mm (2.5 mm through the OMC) |
| Increments | Contiguous, i.e. 5 mm (2.5 mm through the OMC) |
| Scan images | 18–20 |
| Window | Width: 4000 Level +350 |
| Radiation | 120 kV, 100 mA |

OMC, ostiomeatal complex.
*Lund et al. (2000).

Table **8.2**  Radiological staging (Lund–Mackay system 1993).

| Sinus system | Left | Right |
|---|---|---|
| Maxillary (0,1,2) | | |
| Anterior ethmoids (0,1,2) | | |
| Posterior ethmoids (0,1,2) | | |
| Sphenoid (0,1,2) | | |
| Frontal (0,1,2) | | |
| Ostiomeatal complex (0 or 2 only)* | | |
| Total points | | |

0, no abnormalities; 1, partial opacification; 2, total opacification.
*0, not occluded; 2, occluded.

Box 8.1    Anatomical features to be evaluated on CT scan.

Frontal and anterior ethmoid sinuses

　pneumatization of bullae
　frontonasal recess – configuration, e.g. suprabullar cell encroaching on
　frontonasal recess
　lamina papyracea – dehiscence
　roof – height and angle on each side, lateral lamella of cribriform niche,
　dehiscence, angle of crista galli, position of anterior ethmoidal artery
　frontal sinus – size, shape, septa (intersinus and lateral)

Maxillary sinus

　size and shape
　width of infundibulum
　uncinate process
　infraorbital ethmoidal (Haller) cells
　nasolacrimal duct

Posterior ethmoids

　pneumatization with respect to sphenoid, e.g. sphenoethmoidal (Onodi) cells
　and relation to optic nerve

Sphenoid sinus

　optic nerve
　carotid artery

Unfortunately there is no correlation between the many anatomical variants and extent of disease and it should be noted that a significant degree of incidental change can be found in around a third of 'normal' adult controls and in about 45% of children probably related to recent viral upper respiratory tract infections.

CT scans provide information about the extent of mucosal disease, but this correlates poorly with symptoms, surgical findings and histopathology. They also provide useful clues in the diagnosis of atypical sinus infections, such as allergic fungal rhinosinusitis, where chelation of metals by the fungus can lead to an intense or heterogenous signal in the opacified sinuses (Figures 8.6, 8.7) As with skin prick tests the imaging result should be interpreted in the light of the history: in a patient with facial pain at the time of a normal CT scan the diagnosis is unlikely to be sinusitis.

MRI is of help in differentiating various soft tissues from fluid and air, with bone shown as a signal void. The sinonasal mucosa has an excellent blood supply and as a consequence readily gives a high signal which may be confused with inflammatory change. Similarly previous minor upper respiratory tract infections may produce longstanding changes in the sinus mucosa leading to overdiagnosis of disease. Consequently, MRI is reserved, in particular, for the assessment of sinonasal malignancies in combination with CT. Our protocol is shown in Box 8.2. Using this protocol the extent of local tumour spread may be determined with a degree of accuracy in excess of 98% but the final determinant of penetration of the dura and orbital periosteum requires peroperative frozen section assessment.

---

Box 8.2    Imaging protocol for preoperative and postoperative investigation of sinonasal malignancy.*

Pre-operative CT scanning

    direct coronal, axial (one plane with and without contrast enhancement)
    filters and reconstruction algorithms should be suitable for both soft tissue and bone window settings

Preoperative MRI

    coronal, axial and sagittal T1 ($\pm$ gadolinium-DTPA)
    axial T2 – weighted sequence

Postoperative MRI

    coronal, axial and sagittal T1 pre and post-gadolinium-DTPA with subtraction
    axial T2-weighted sequence

---

* Lloyd et al 2000

Imaging, in particular MRI, also plays an important role in the post-therapeutic follow up of patients with sinonasal tumours indicating areas of residual or recurrent disease and defining suspicious areas for biopsy.

## References

Lloyd GAS, Lund VJ, Howard DJ, Savy L (2000) Optimum imaging for sinonasal malignancy, *J Laryngol Otol* **114**: 557–62.

Lund VJ, Mackay IS (1993) Staging in rhinosinusitis, *Rhinology* **31**: 183–4

Lund VJ, Savy G, Lloyd GAS (2000) Optimum Imaging for Endoscopic Sinus Surgery in Adults, *J Laryngol Otol* **114**: 395–7.

## Further reading

Jones NS (2000) CT of the paranasal sinuses: a review of the correlation with clinical, surgical and histopathological findings, *Clin Otol* **27**: 11–17.

Lloyd GA, Lund VJ, Scadding GK (1991) CT of the paranasal sinuses and functional endoscopic sinus surgery: a critical analysis of 100 symptomatic patients, *J Laryngol Otol* **105**: 181–5.

Lund VJ, Kennedy DW (1995) Quantification for staging rhinosinusitis. The staging and therapy group, *Ann Otol Rhinol Laryngol Suppl* **167**: 17–21.

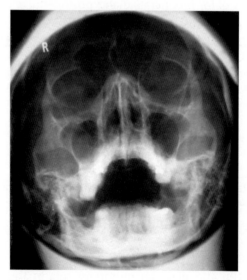

Figure **8.1**

Plain sinus x-ray – occipito-mental view showing some mucosal thickening in the right maxillary antrum.

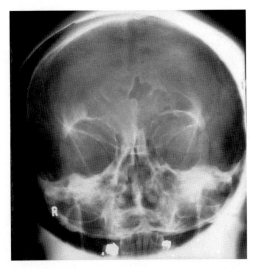

Figure **8.2**

Plain sinus x-ray – occipito-mental view showing opacification of the frontal sinuses, worse on the right.

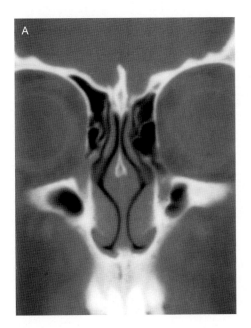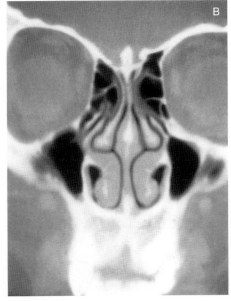

Figure **8.3**

(A) Coronal CT scan of sinuses showing normal anatomy of the anterior middle meatus showing the septal tubercle and nasolacrimal ducts. (B) Coronal CT scan of sinuses showing normal anatomy of the ostiomeatal complex.

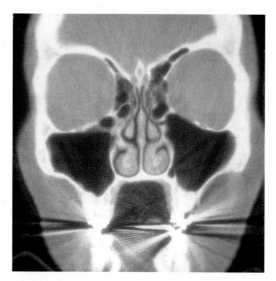

Figure **8.4**

Coronal CT scan showing normal sinuses but crowding of the infundibulum by infra-orbital cells (Haller cells).

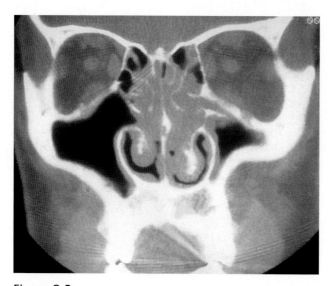

Figure **8.5**

Coronal CT scan showing mucosal thickening in the central nasal cavity extending into the left infundibulum and ethmoids but with peripheral pneumatisation (a black halo).

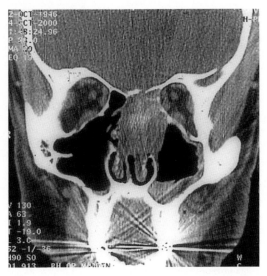

Figure **8.6**

Coronal CT scan showing a unilateral mass in the left upper nasal cavity and posterior ethmoids. Heterogeneity in the secretion strongly suggestive of fungal disease due to the presence of trace elements and heavy metals.

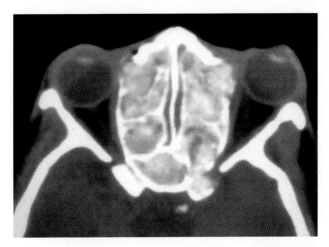

Figure **8.7**

Axial Ct scan showing massive expansion and complete opacification of the ethmoids producing pseudo-hypertelorism. Heterogeneity of the secretion again highly suggestive of allergic fungal rhinosinusitis.

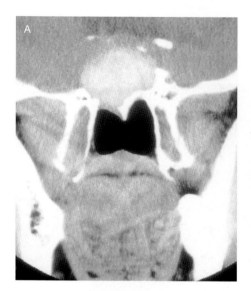
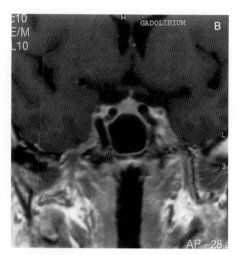

Figure **8.8**

(A) Coronal CT scan showing complete opacification of the sphenoid with marked bone erosion. Heterogeneity of secretion highly suggestive of fungal ball. (B) MRI scan in same patient showing signal void produced by fungal secretion erroneously suggesting an empty sphenoid.

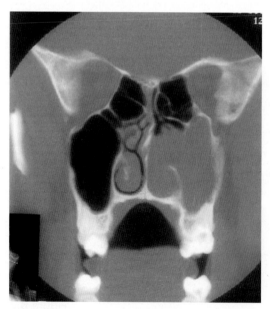

Figure **8.9**

Coronal CT scan showing opacification of the left maxillary antrum and nasal cavity due to an antrochoanal polyp.

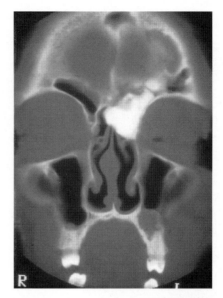

Figure **8.10**

Coronal CT scan showing lobulated dense mass in the right frontal sinus, typical of an osteoma.

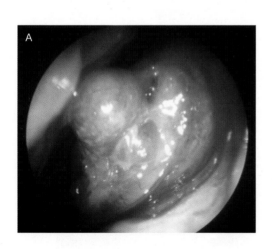

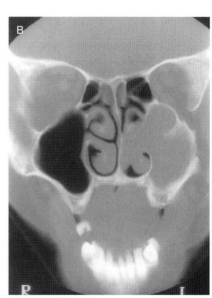

Figure **8.11**

(A) Endoscopic photograph of the middle left meatus showing inverted papilloma. (B) Coronal CT in the same patient showing inverted papilloma in the left maxillary sinus and middle meatus with typical hyperdensity.

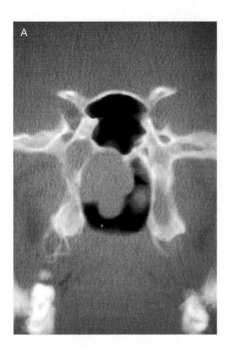

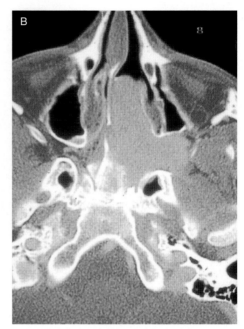

## Figure **8.12**

(A) Coronal CT showing unilateral mass in the posterior choana associated with erosion of the upper medial pterygoid plate, appearances pathognomonic of juvenile angio-fibroma. (B) Axial CT scan in same patient showing mass filling the posterior part of the nasal cavity with expansion of the pterygopalatine fossa, extension into the infra-temporal fossa and anterior displacement of the back wall of the maxillary antrum.

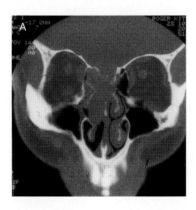

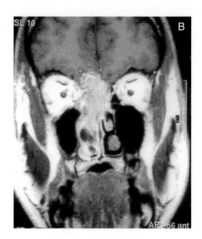

## Figure **8.13**

(A) Coronal CT scan showing unilateral mass of olfactory neuroblastoma in the right upper nasal cavity with associated bony erosion of the skull base. (B) MRI – T1 weighted with gadolinium in same patient showing extension of the mass into the anterior cranial fossa.

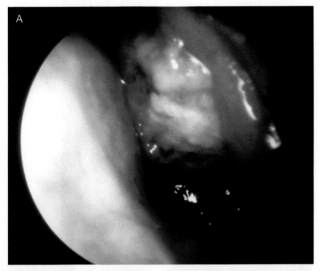

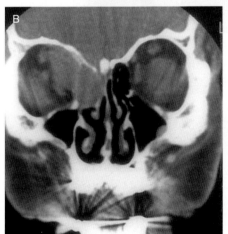

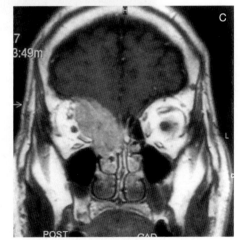

Figure **8.14**

(A) Endoscopic photograph showing malignant melanoma in the right middle meatus. (B) Coronal CT scan in same patient showing tumour affecting the right anterior ethmoids extending into the orbit with thinning of the skull base. (C) Coronal MRI scan (T1 weighted with gadolinium) in same patient.

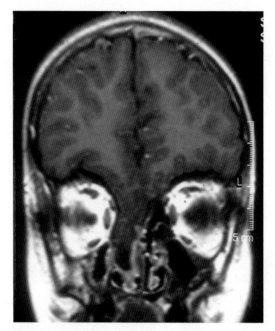

Figure **8.15**

Coronal MRI showing meningocele in upper right nasal cavity.

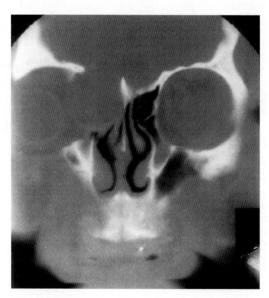

Figure **8.16**

Coronal CT scan showing smooth expansile lesion in the right frontal region, typical of a mucocele.

# 9

# Other tests

## Olfaction

Patients can present with reduced or absent sense of smell for a variety of reasons. An algorithm for investigation is provided in the Appendix

The sense of smell is difficult to test objectively. Olfactory evoked responses have been measured, but are not in routine clinical use. The test most widely used for evaluation is the UPSIT (University of Pennsylvania Smell Identification Test) (Figure 9.1). This has been validated and the format, which involves scratch and sniff testing with forced choice from four possible answers for each odour, allows differentiation of malingerers. The result is given as the number of smells correctly identified out of 40 and the patient is assigned to normosmia, hyposmia or anosmia according to age based on a graph derived from hundreds of subjects. Unfortunately, the UPSIT test is expensive, has to be imported and contains many odours

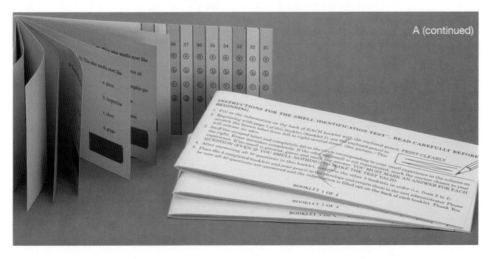

Figure **9.1**

The University of Pennsylvania Smell Identification Test (UPSIT) booklets, each containing 10 patches.

B

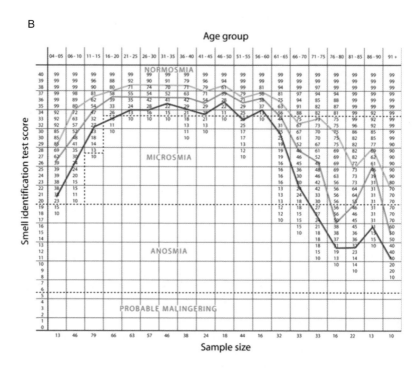

C

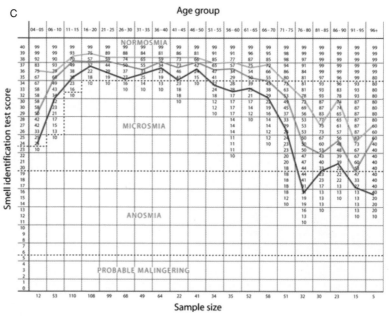

Figure **9.1** Continued

Normative data for UPSIT results in (B) males and (C) females

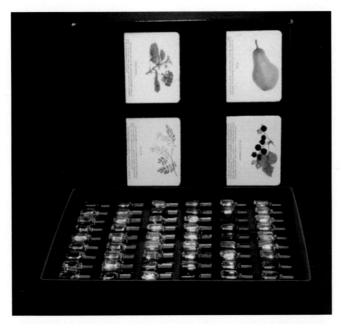

Figure **9.2**

The Nez du Vin – a set of odours designed to educate wine tasters.

which are specifically American, thus very few patients in the United Kingdom score full marks.

Alternative tests have been devised. Among these is the Nez du Vin (Figure 9.2) which involves six odours and again a forced choice between four possibilities for each. This has been shown to correlate with the UPSIT test and can be used to screen patients: those scoring five or six are regarded as normosmic. Similar tests are commercially available. A Swiss version has the advantage of picture identification so that language is not a barrier.

Threshold testing can also be undertaken using pm-carbinol (Figure 9.3) in commercially prepared dilutions. The patient is asked to differentiate between the real substance in various dilutions against a blank preparation.

When undertaking tests of smell the patient should also have their nasal airway examined and measured. It is customary to test taste at the same time. This involves solutions of glucose, citric acid, quinine and sodium chloride with sweet, sour, bitter and salty tastes respectively. One drop is placed on the tongue and the subject has to describe the taste. The mouth should be rinsed with water between tests. It is very rare for the sense of taste to be completely lost since the nerve supply to the tongue is duplicated.

A

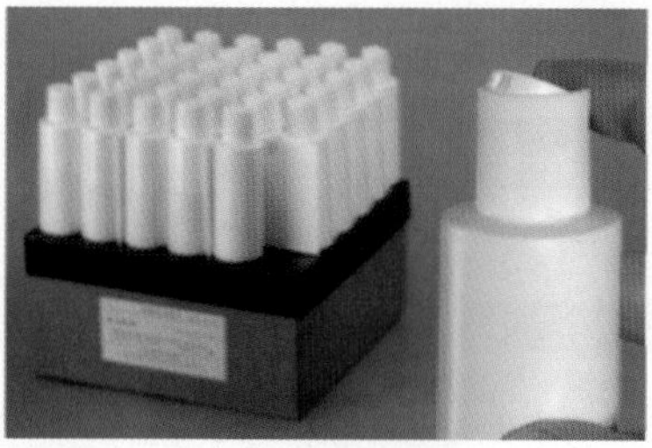

B

SPECIFIC ANOSMIA TESTS

Test odor level = 25 dS (18 x mean threshold, or +2 S.D.)

Name:_____ Sex:_____ Age:____

Ethnic:_____ Cigs. per day:____

Tester:_____ Place:_____ Date: __/__/__

Days since start of last menses:___ Months of pregnancy:___

Any smell or taste problems?

To avoid contaminating the bottles, and for an accurate test
result, it is essential that the following answers are "No":-

Has Subject   smoked in the   last 15 min.?____
Any food, drink or candy in last 15 min.?____
Any odor or perfume on the hands or face?____
Any sign of a nasal infection or allergy?____
Are there odors at Subject's  work-place?____
Any odors in the area used for this test?____

| NO. | LABEL | DESCRIPTION; COMMENT | 1st | 2nd | 3rd | S/N |
|-----|-------|---------------------|-----|-----|-----|-----|
| 1 | IV-ACID | | | | | |
| 2 | TM-AMINE | | | | | |
| 3 | ANDROSTONE | | | | | |
| 4 | PD-LACTONE | | | | | |
| 5 | L-CARVONE | | | | | |
| 6 | CINEOLE | | | | | |
| 7 | TB-THIOL | | | | | |
| 8 | PE-ALCOHOL | | | | | |
| 9 | MH-ACID | | | | | |
| 10 | MI-BORNEOL | | | | | |
| 11 | DIACETYL | | | | | |
| 12 | THIOPHANE | | | | | |

Explanation (see over):

Figure 9.3

(A) The pm-carbinol threshold test kit. (B) Test chart for specific anosmia.

# Testing for cerebrospinal fluid (CSF)

Rhinorrhoea which is unilateral or which occurs mainly on rising in the morning and bending forward suggests the possibility of a cerebrospinal fluid (CSF) leak. Accurate diagnosis of this condition has been improved by non-invasive electrophoretic testing of nasal secretions for beta2-transferrin (asialotransferrin) which is found practically only in CSF and not in other body fluids. The high specificity and sensitivity of the test depend on the fact that the low sialic acid content of beta2-transferrin delays its mobility in electrophoretic gels compared to that of beta1-transferrin. Even under unfavourable conditions, 10% CSF can be detected. The test takes about 5 hours, uses 110 minutes of operator time and costs between €150–300. However, it can save unnecessary invasive investigations or surgery. As a negative result means that the fluid is not CSF.

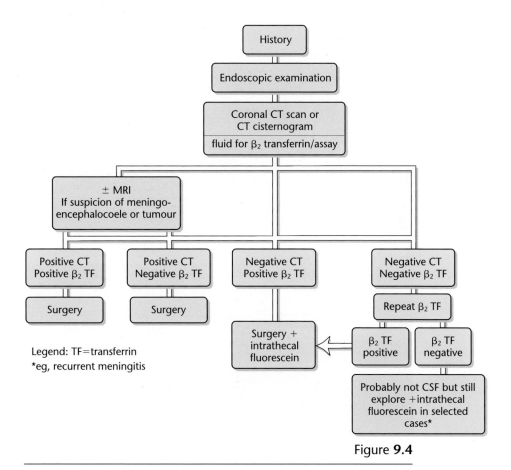

Figure **9.4**

Algorithm for the management of CSF rhinorrhoea.
Reproduced with permission of the Editor, Journal of Laryngology and Otology

## Nasal biopsy

Histological diagnosis of rhinitis is rarely required. Nasal biopsies are frequently unhelpful in patients with suspected granulomatous or vasculitic disease, tending to show only non-specific inflammatory changes and often being complicated by haemorrhage, even when taken at obviously involved sites. However, in suspected allergic fungal rhinosinusitis all material should be sent to the laboratory with instructions for specific fungal stains such as Grocott's. This may show only a few hyphae with a massive inflammatory response. Fungal culture is of no help in diagnosis since fungi can be cultured from practically all noses. Similarly, all polyps should undergo histological examination, certainly on first removal, in case there is a rare underlying malignancy. Nasal biopsy has proved useful in elucidating the mechanisms of allergic and non-allergic rhinitis. Gerritsma forceps which have a cup that collects the pinhead-sized specimen are ideal for this purpose.

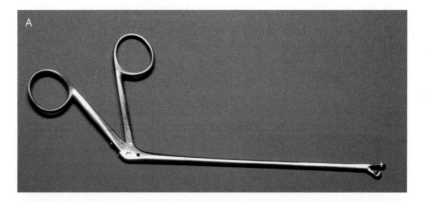

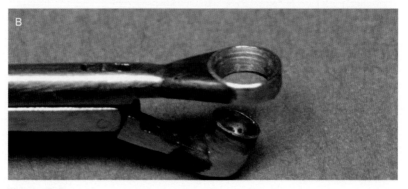

Figure **9.5**

(A) Gerritsma forceps. (B) Close up of cup which collects biopsy specimen.

# Microbiology

Nasal swabs are invariably infected with multiple organisms since the nose is not sterile. If an attempt is to be made in the clinic to find the infecting organism in rhinosinusitis then a middle meatal swab has to be taken using the endoscope to guide the procedure. Studies comparing such results to those taken peroperatively from the sinuses suggest good correlation. Sinus swabs are useful in immune deficient patients, especially those on prophylactic antibiotics, to guide further therapy. The significance of the result to treatment need is debatable in non-immunodeficient patients in whom rhinosinusitis may be inflammatory rather than primarily infective.

# Quality of life

The recent appreciation that rhinosinusitis has marked effects upon quality of life has led to inclusion of such instruments in therapeutic trials. Generic measures include the short form 36 (SF36) which can be used to compare values across different diseases.

Specific instruments include the RLQL and SNOT 20. (see Appendix).

All of these can be filled in by the patient whilst waiting in the clinic after brief explanation. All have the disadvantage that other life events can alter symptom perception.

# Further reading

Amoore JE, Ollman BG (1983). Practical test kits for quantitatively evaluating the sense of smell, *Rhinology* **21**: 49–54.

Arrer E, Gibitz HJ (1987). Detection of beta-2 transferrin with agarose gel electrophoresis, immunofixation and silver staining in cerebrospinal fluid, secretions and other body fluids, *J Clin Chem Clin Biochem* **25**: 113–16.

Lund VJ (2002) Endoscopic management of CSF leaks, *Am J Rhinol* **16**: 17–23.

# Appendix 1

## Oral allergy syndrome

This condition is usually caused by sensitivity to certain fresh fruits and vegetables. Most sufferers have other allergies in addition, most usually to certain pollens. In a few sufferers the condition may be associated with a true allergy to other foods such as shrimp or egg, and for these the risk of a more severe generalized reaction is greater. However, in the most common form, sufferers who are allergic to certain pollens also experience a localized swelling or itching of the lips, mouth, tongue or throat immediately after contact with certain fruits or vegetables. Reactions usually follow contact with the fresh fruit or raw vegetable, although reactions to cooked foods can sometimes also occur.

### Pollens involved

A number of pollen allergies may be connected with the condition, although the commonest related allergy is to birch pollen. It has been estimated that as many as 75% of birch-allergic patients may be affected, although those with the mildest form (a sensation in the lips or tongue after eating raw apples) may not have realized that there was an allergic problem. Other pollens involved include grass, daisy family and certain weeds.

Adults appear to develop this condition more often than children, local reaction to fruits and vegetables being the most frequently encountered source of true (immediate) food allergy in sufferers over the age of 10. Children appear more likely to suffer generalized allergic reactions (e.g. rash, vomiting or wheeze) as a response to foods to which they are allergic.

### Symptoms

These symptoms may occur:

- Redness, swelling and itching, with or without rash (blotchy, pimply or even blistering) of lips, tongue, inside of mouth and soft palate.

| Plant material | Cross-reacting foods | |
|----------------|---------------------|---|
| Silver birch pollen | Almond | Mango |
| | Aniseed | Nectarine |
| | Apple (raw) | Onion (raw) |
| | Apricot | Orange |
| | Caraway | Parsley |
| | Carrot (raw) | Peach |
| | Celery (raw) | Pepper (capsicum) |
| | Cherry | Plum |
| | Coriander | Potato (raw) |
| | Hazelnut | Tomato (raw) |
| | Kiwi | Walnut |
| | Lychee | |
| Grass pollen | Kiwi | Tomato (raw) |
| | Melon | Watermelon |
| | Peanut | Wheat |
| Daisy family pollens | Lychee | Sunflower seeds |
| Mugwort (weed) pollen | Aniseed | Fennel |
| | Carrot (raw) | Parsley |
| | Celery (raw) | Spices (some) |
| | Celery salt | |
| Latex (contact and/or inhaled allergy | Avocado | Papaya |
| | Banana | Peach |
| | Chestnut | Peppers |
| | Kiwi | Pineapple |
| | Mango | Plum |
| | Melon | Tomato (raw) |
| | Orange | |

Oral allergy syndrome associated plant allergens and their cross-reacting food allergens. Patients generally react to some *but not all* foods in a particular group, and should only avoid those giving symptoms.

- Occasionally itchy swelling of the throat may occur (celery is a particular culprit).
- Symptoms in the oesophagus (gullet) or stomach include pain and discomfort, heartburn, nausea and even vomiting.
- General symptoms such as urticaria (nettle rash), rhinitis and asthma may occur after an interval, particularly if the sufferer ignores the local symptoms and eats all of the culprit food.
- Very rarely anaphylactic shock (allergic collapse) may occur (e.g. peanut, almond, apricot and peach).

## Reaction clusters

Certain food reactions commonly occur together. These may be called food 'clusters'. Allergy to particular pollen is commonly found for those who react to each food cluster. Allergy to latex (the plant material from which rubber is produced) is also found to cross-react with certain plant allergens so that some sufferers may react to both skin contact with latex (e.g. balloons, rubber gloves, elastic, many medical devices) and oral contact with certain foods.

Some foods seem only to cause problems when eaten in the raw state (often the case with carrot and apple) and eating the foods when cooked causes no problem.

## Treatment

The correct identification and subsequent avoidance of the culprit food or foods must be the first objective. Previous experience of what has happened in the past when eating certain foods is the most important evidence. Skin and blood tests can help to confirm the diagnosis. It does not follow that all the foods of a particular group will cause trouble for a sufferer who reacts to one or two of them, only the foods that have caused symptoms in the past should be avoided.

In an occasional case where it is considered that there may be a small risk of severe or generalized reaction a sufferer may be advised to carry epinephrine by injection as a precaution. In other cases an epinephrine spray (for the mouth and throat) may be advised.

Most sufferers have mild symptoms and can generally be reassured that their condition is never likely to become severe, although it is unlikely that they will ever grow out of it. Desensitization treatment for this condition is not available at the present time.

# Appendix 2

## A guide for aspirin-sensitive patients

**Dangerous drugs:** People known to be aspirin-sensitive must not take aspirin or drug products containing aspirin or aspirin-like drugs (see below), which are usually used for rheumatism, pain or fever.

---

**Common drugs containing aspirin**

Alka-Seltzer  Analgesic Dellipsoids D6  Anodyne Dellipsoids D4  Antoin  APC Mixture  Asagran  Aspav  Aspellin  Broprin  Caprin  Claradin  Co-Codaprin  Codis  Dolasan  Doloxene Co  Equagesic  Hypon  Laboprin  Levius  Migravess  Myolgin  Napsalgesic  Nu-Seals Aspirin  Onadox 118  Paynocil  Robaxisal Forte  Safapryn  Safapryn Co  Solprin  Sore Throat Mixture  Trancoprin  Veganin

---

**Common aspirin-like drugs (NSAIDs)**

Alrheumat  Apsifen  Artracin  Benoral  Brufen  Butacote  Bulazolidin  Disalcid  Dolobid  Ebutac  Flinoril  Feldene  Fenbid Spansule  Feno-pron  Froben  Ibumetin  Ibuprofen  Imbrilon  Indocid  Indoflex  Indolar  Indomod  Iorunvail  Laraflex  Larapam  Lederfen  Lodine  Motrin  Naprosyn  Nurofen  Orudis  Oruvail  Palaprin Forte  Paxofen  Ponstan  Progesic  Ramodar  Relifex  Rheumox  Surgam  Synflex  Tolectin  Voltarol

---

● **Important: As the list cannot ever be complete, make sure that any drug you take does not contain aspirin or aspirin-like drugs by looking at the label. If in doubt ask your chemist.**

### Salicylates, drugs and food chemicals

If you have a salicylate intolerance, it is possible that you may also react to aspirin, and that any drug containing aspirin or aspirin-like drugs will be likely to affect you. However intolerance of salicylates may also be associated with intolerance of other chemicals, dyes

**Common dyes (E numbers)**

Tartrazine (102) Yellow 2G (107) Sunset yellow – cordials/custards (110) Amaranth (123) Ponceau 4R – red berry/cherry flavours/jellies (124) Brilliant Black – blackcurrant flavours/sauces (151) Brown HT – chocolate flavourings/sauces (155)

**Common preservatives**

Benzoates – fruit juice/drinks (210, 211, 212, 213)
Sulphites – wine/sausages/fruit juices/flours/pickles (220, 221, 222, 223, 224, 225, 228)
Gallates (antioxidants) – oils and fats (310, 311, 312)

and preservatives (see above). These may also need to be avoided. In general use fresh and home-made foods rather than prepared ones.

## Foods containing salicylates

In addition some aspirin-sensitive individuals react to foods containing salicylates. All fresh meat, fish, shellfish, poultry, eggs, dairy products, cereals and bread are low in salicylates. See below for a breakdown on type and levels of salicylates in various foods.

**Vegetables**

**Low** – bamboo shoots bean sprouts brussel sprouts red cabbage green cabbage celery chickpeas chives choko kidney beans leeks lentils lettuce lima beans fresh peas dried peas peeled potatoes shallots swedes

**Moderate** – asparagus beans green beetroot carrots cauliflowers kumera marrows mushrooms onions parsnips unpeeled potato pumpkins sweetcorn turnips

**High** – alfalfa sprouts broad beans broccoli cucumbers eggplant spinach watercress

**Very high** – capsicums courgettes gherkins olives radishes tomato and tomato-based foods potato skins

**Fruits**

**Low** – Golden Delicious apples  bananas  peeled pears  paw-paws

**Moderate** – Red Delicious apples  grapefruits  kiwifruits  lemons  mangoes  passion fruit  pears with skin  persimmon  rhubarb  tamarillo  watermelons

**High** – Granny Smith apples  gala apples  cherries  lychees  mandarins  peaches

**Very high** – apricots  berry fruits  grapes  oranges  plums  pineapples  rock melon  all dried fruit (sultanas  raisins  prunes  dates etc.)  all jams  jellies  marmalades  fruit juices

**Other foods**

**Low** – garlic  parsley  soy sauce  malt vinegar  cashew nuts  poppy  seeds  cocoa  carob  sugar  golden syrup  chocolate  camomile tea  dandelion coffee  tonic water  gin  vodka  whisky

**Moderate** – nuts  coconut  sesame seeds  sunflower seeds  beer  cider  sherry  brandy

**High** – honey  marmite  vegemite  coffee  wine  port  fruit teas

**Very high** – herbs and spices (e.g. curry powder, oregano, turmeric)  white vinegar  Worcester sauce  tea  peppermint tea  rum  liqueurs

To test this out stick to low foods for a 2-week period, then try adding in moderate foods again for 2 weeks. If no worse test out high foods in the same way and then the very high. Please report any reactions.

# Appendix 3

## Quality of Life Instruments

### Rhinitis quality of life questionnaire

This exists in 3 forms: original, standardised and mini. It is obtainable from its originator, Elizabeth Juniper, free of charge to all clinicians and at juniper@qoltech.co.uk or Elizabeth Juniper, MCSP, MSc. 20 Marcuse Fields, Bosham, West Sussex, PO18 8NA, England.

Further information, e.g. about the languages in which the questionnaires are available, can be found at www.qoltech.co.uk

### SNOT-20

This can be found at www.oto.wust1.edu/clinepi/Forms/inst_shot. 20.doc. Its originator, Jay Piccirillo, is glad to provide copies to investigators who wish to use it for academic research.

Dr. J. Piccirillo, Washington University School of Medicine, Clinical Outcomes Research Office Department of Otolaryngology, 660 South Euclid Ave. Campus Box 8115, St. Louis, MO (314) 362-7394 World Wide Web: http://oto.wustl.edu/clinepi

## Instructions for Scoring SNOT-20

*Patient rates the severity of their condition on each of the 20 items such as 'need to blow the nose', 'wake up at night', using a 0–5 category rating system:*

0 = Not present/no problem
1 = Very mild problem
2 = Mild or slight problem
3 = Moderate problem
4 = Severe problem
5 = Problem as "bad as it can be"

Next, the patient identifies the most important items to them and the items they hope will improve the most with treatment (up to a maximum of 5 items)

## SNOT-20 Scoring:

- The Total SNOT-20 score is calculated as the mean item score for all 20 items
- The possible range of SNOT-20 score is 0–5, with higher scores indicating greater rhinosinusitis-related health burden
- The SNOT-20 Change Score is the difference between Pre-treatment and Post-treatment Total SNOT-20 score
- Impact of treatment is assessed with the SNOT-20 Change Score
- A separate SNOT-20 score and Change score is also calculated based on the items rated as Important.

# Appendix 4

A. Form for a paediatric patient

B. Form for an adult patient

C. Form for middle ear dysfunction

A

## Paediatric Rhinitis Clinic

PLEASE FILL IN AS FULLY AND ACCURATELY AS POSSIBLE AND BRING WITH YOU TO THE CLINIC

Child's Surname . . . . . . . . . . . . . . . . . . . . . . . . . . . . . . . . . . .

First Names . . . . . . . . . . . . . . . . . . . . . . . . . . . . . . . . . . . . . .

Date of Birth . . . . . . . . . . . . . . . . . . . . . . . . . . . . . . . . . . . . .

Address . . . . . . . . . . . . . . . . . . . . . . . . . . . . . . . . . . . . . . . . .

. . . . . . . . . . . . . . . . . . . . . . . . . . . . . . . . . . . . . . . . . . . . . .

. . . . . . . . . . . . . . . . . . . . . . . . . . . . . . . . . . . . . . . . . . . . . .

. . . . . . . . . . . . . . . . . . . . . . . . . . . . . . . . . . . . . . . . . . . . . .

Telephone Number . . . . . . . . . . . . . . . . . . . . . . . . . . . . . . . . .

N.H.S. Number . . . . . . . . . . . . . . . . . . . . . . . . . . . . . . . . . . . .

What is the main reason for referral to the clinic? . . . . . . . . . . . . . .

. . . . . . . . . . . . . . . . . . . . . . . . . . . . . . . . . . . . . . . . . . . . . .

. . . . . . . . . . . . . . . . . . . . . . . . . . . . . . . . . . . . . . . . . . . . . .

Are there any other problems or difficulties which may be relevant? . .

. . . . . . . . . . . . . . . . . . . . . . . . . . . . . . . . . . . . . . . . . . . . . .

. . . . . . . . . . . . . . . . . . . . . . . . . . . . . . . . . . . . . . . . . . . . . .

. . . . . . . . . . . . . . . . . . . . . . . . . . . . . . . . . . . . . . . . . . . . . .

**Please circle any of the following which apply to your child:**

Running nose

Clear nasal discharge

Thick nasal discharge, often green/yellow

Sneezing

Blocked nose          left side          right side          both sides

Snoring

Mouth breathing at night

Itchy nose

Rubs nose with fingers/hand

Lacks sense of smell

Lacks sense of taste

When did these symptoms start? . . . . . . . . . . . . . . . . . . . . . . . . . . .

. . . . . . . . . . . . . . . . . . . . . . . . . . . . . . . . . . . . . . . . . . . . . . . . . . . . .

. . . . . . . . . . . . . . . . . . . . . . . . . . . . . . . . . . . . . . . . . . . . . . . . . . . . .

Are they worse at any particular time of year?　　　　Yes / No

If so, when? . . . . . . . . . . . . . . . . . . . . . . . . . . . . . . . . . . . . . . . . . . . .

. . . . . . . . . . . . . . . . . . . . . . . . . . . . . . . . . . . . . . . . . . . . . . . . . . . . .

Are they worse at any particular time of day?　　　　Yes / No

If so, when? . . . . . . . . . . . . . . . . . . . . . . . . . . . . . . . . . . . . . . . . . . . .

. . . . . . . . . . . . . . . . . . . . . . . . . . . . . . . . . . . . . . . . . . . . . . . . . . . . .

Is there anything that you know of which will make the
symptoms worse?　　　　Yes / No

If so, what? . . . . . . . . . . . . . . . . . . . . . . . . . . . . . . . . . . . . . . . . . . . . .

. . . . . . . . . . . . . . . . . . . . . . . . . . . . . . . . . . . . . . . . . . . . . . . . . . . . .

. . . . . . . . . . . . . . . . . . . . . . . . . . . . . . . . . . . . . . . . . . . . . . . . . . . . .

. . . . . . . . . . . . . . . . . . . . . . . . . . . . . . . . . . . . . . . . . . . . . . . . . . . . .

Are they worse in any particular place?　　　　Yes / No

If so, where? . . . . . . . . . . . . . . . . . . . . . . . . . . . . . . . . . . . . . . . . . . . .

. . . . . . . . . . . . . . . . . . . . . . . . . . . . . . . . . . . . . . . . . . . . . . . . . . . . .

. . . . . . . . . . . . . . . . . . . . . . . . . . . . . . . . . . . . . . . . . . . . . . . . . . . . .

. . . . . . . . . . . . . . . . . . . . . . . . . . . . . . . . . . . . . . . . . . . . . . . . . . . . .

A

Does your child

Wheeze?                                                          Yes / No

Get out of breath easily?                                        Yes / No

Have a frequent dry cough?                                       Yes / No

Cough at night?                                                  Yes / No

Suffer from frequent chest infections?                           Yes / No

Suffer from frequent ear infections?                             Yes / No

Have a lot of sore throats                                       Yes / No

Have difficulty in hearing?                                      Yes / No

Do you think your child was/is late in talking?                  Yes / No

Do you think your child is difficult to
understand?                                          Yes / No / Sometimes

**Birth History**

Was the pregnancy normal?                                        Yes / No

If not, please specify what problems occurred . . . . . . . . . . . . . . . . . .

. . . . . . . . . . . . . . . . . . . . . . . . . . . . . . . . . . . . . . . . . . . . . . . . .

. . . . . . . . . . . . . . . . . . . . . . . . . . . . . . . . . . . . . . . . . . . . . . . . .

| Labour | Normal | Rapid | Prolonged | |
|---|---|---|---|---|
| Delivery | Normal | Forceps | Breech | Caesarian |

Full term                                                        Yes / No

If not, at how many weeks? . . . . . . . . . . . . . . . . . . . . . . . . . . . . . . .

Birth weight . . . . . . . . . . . . . . . . . . . . . . lb/oz

. . . . . . . . . . . . . . . . . . . . . . . . . . . . . . kg

Condition at birth

Normal                    Difficulty with breathing                    Jaundice

**Feeding**

Breastfed?                                                    Yes / No

If so, for how long? . . . . . . . . . . . . . . . . . . . . . . . . . . . . . . . . . . . . . .

Bottle-fed?                                                   Yes / No

When was bottled milk first given? . . . . . . . . . . . . . . . . . . . . . . . . . . .

Type of milk used . . . . . . . . . . . . . . . . . . . . . . . . . . . . . . . . . . . . . . . .

Did the baby feed well?                                      Yes / No

If not, what problems occurred . . . . . . . . . . . . . . . . . . . . . . . . . . . . . .

. . . . . . . . . . . . . . . . . . . . . . . . . . . . . . . . . . . . . . . . . . . . . . . . . . . . . . .

. . . . . . . . . . . . . . . . . . . . . . . . . . . . . . . . . . . . . . . . . . . . . . . . . . . . . . .

Any colic?                                                   Yes / No

When was weaning first started? . . . . . . . . . . . . . . . . . . . . . . . . . . . . .

Which foods were introduced? . . . . . . . . . . . . . . . . . . . . . . . . . . . . . .

. . . . . . . . . . . . . . . . . . . . . . . . . . . . . . . . . . . . . . . . . . . . . . . . . . . . . . .

Has your baby suffered from any severe illnesses?           Yes / No

Which? . . . . . . . . . . . . . . . . . . . . . . . . . . . . . . . . . . . . . . . . . . . . . . . . .

Has your child had any operations?                          Yes / No

Nature of operation(s) and date(s) . . . . . . . . . . . . . . . . . . . . . . . . . . .

. . . . . . . . . . . . . . . . . . . . . . . . . . . . . . . . . . . . . . . . . . . . . . . . . . . . . . .

. . . . . . . . . . . . . . . . . . . . . . . . . . . . . . . . . . . . . . . . . . . . . . . . . . . . . . .

**Family History**

Are there any other children in the family?                 Yes / No

Please give the age and sex of each one . . . . . . . . . . . . . . . . . . . . . . .

. . . . . . . . . . . . . . . . . . . . . . . . . . . . . . . . . . . . . . . . . . . . . . . . . . . . . . .

. . . . . . . . . . . . . . . . . . . . . . . . . . . . . . . . . . . . . . . . . . . . . . . . . . . . . . .

A

Does anyone in the family have allergies?                    Yes / No
(Asthma, eczema, hay fever, urticaria, food allergy, drug allergy etc.)

Please specify . . . . . . . . . . . . . . . . . . . . . . . . . . . . . . . . . . . . . . . .

. . . . . . . . . . . . . . . . . . . . . . . . . . . . . . . . . . . . . . . . . . . . . . . . . .

. . . . . . . . . . . . . . . . . . . . . . . . . . . . . . . . . . . . . . . . . . . . . . . . . .

Does anyone in the family suffer from repeated infections?    Yes / No

Please specify . . . . . . . . . . . . . . . . . . . . . . . . . . . . . . . . . . . . . . . .

. . . . . . . . . . . . . . . . . . . . . . . . . . . . . . . . . . . . . . . . . . . . . . . . . .

**Potential Allergens**

Please tick any of the following which are in your home:

| Carpets | Mould | Feather/down Duvet |
|---|---|---|
| Central Heating | Trees | Wool Blankets |
| Pets | Furry Toys | Cigarette Smoke |
| Damp | Feather Pillows | |

**Diet**

Any food fads or fancies?                                  Yes / No

If so, please specify . . . . . . . . . . . . . . . . . . . . . . . . . . . . . . . . . . . .

. . . . . . . . . . . . . . . . . . . . . . . . . . . . . . . . . . . . . . . . . . . . . . . . . .

. . . . . . . . . . . . . . . . . . . . . . . . . . . . . . . . . . . . . . . . . . . . . . . . . .

Does your child eat a lot of dairy products?                Yes / No

Does your child eat a lot of junk food?                     Yes / No

Do any foods upset your child?                              Yes / No

## Medications

What treatments has your child tried? . . . . . . . . . . . . . . . . . . . . . . .

. . . . . . . . . . . . . . . . . . . . . . . . . . . . . . . . . . . . . . . . . . . . . . .

Has your child ever reacted to medicine?                    Yes / No

Please specify . . . . . . . . . . . . . . . . . . . . . . . . . . . . . . . . . . . . . . .

. . . . . . . . . . . . . . . . . . . . . . . . . . . . . . . . . . . . . . . . . . . . . . .

Which, if any, have proved helpful? . . . . . . . . . . . . . . . . . . . . . . . .

. . . . . . . . . . . . . . . . . . . . . . . . . . . . . . . . . . . . . . . . . . . . . . .

## Adult Rhinitis Clinic

PLEASE FILL IN AS FULLY AND ACCURATELY AS POSSIBLE AND BRING WITH YOU TO THE CLINIC

Surname . . . . . . . . . . . . . . . . . . . . . . . . . . . . . . . . . . . . . . . . . . . . .

First Names . . . . . . . . . . . . . . . . . . . . . . . . . . . . . . . . . . . . . . . . . .

Date of Birth . . . . . . . . . . . . . . . . . . . . . . . . . . . . . . . . . . . . . . . . .

Address . . . . . . . . . . . . . . . . . . . . . . . . . . . . . . . . . . . . . . . . . . . . .

. . . . . . . . . . . . . . . . . . . . . . . . . . . . . . . . . . . . . . . . . . . . . . . . . . .

. . . . . . . . . . . . . . . . . . . . . . . . . . . . . . . . . . . . . . . . . . . . . . . . . . .

. . . . . . . . . . . . . . . . . . . . . . . . . . . . . . . . . . . . . . . . . . . . . . . . . . .

Telephone Number . . . . . . . . . . . . . . . . . . . . . . . . . . . . . . . . . . . .

Occupation . . . . . . . . . . . . . . . . . . . . . . . . . . . . . . . . . . . . . . . . . .

What is the main reason for referral to the clinic? . . . . . . . . . . . . . . .

. . . . . . . . . . . . . . . . . . . . . . . . . . . . . . . . . . . . . . . . . . . . . . . . . . .

. . . . . . . . . . . . . . . . . . . . . . . . . . . . . . . . . . . . . . . . . . . . . . . . . . .

Are there any other problems or difficulties which may be relevant? . .

. . . . . . . . . . . . . . . . . . . . . . . . . . . . . . . . . . . . . . . . . . . . . . . . . . .

. . . . . . . . . . . . . . . . . . . . . . . . . . . . . . . . . . . . . . . . . . . . . . . . . . .

. . . . . . . . . . . . . . . . . . . . . . . . . . . . . . . . . . . . . . . . . . . . . . . . . . .

**Please circle any of the following which apply to you:**

Running nose

Clear nasal discharge

Thick nasal discharge, often green/yellow

Sneezing

Blocked nose          left side          right side          both sides

Snoring

Mouth breathing at night

Itchy nose

Rub nose with fingers/hand

Lack sense of smell

Lack sense of taste

When did these symptoms start? . . . . . . . . . . . . . . . . . . . . . . . . . . .

. . . . . . . . . . . . . . . . . . . . . . . . . . . . . . . . . . . . . . . . . . . . . . . . . . . . .

. . . . . . . . . . . . . . . . . . . . . . . . . . . . . . . . . . . . . . . . . . . . . . . . . . . . .

Are they worse at any particular time of year?          Yes  /  No

If so, when? . . . . . . . . . . . . . . . . . . . . . . . . . . . . . . . . . . . . . . . . .

. . . . . . . . . . . . . . . . . . . . . . . . . . . . . . . . . . . . . . . . . . . . . . . . . . . . .

Are they worse at any particular time of day?           Yes  /  No

If so, when? . . . . . . . . . . . . . . . . . . . . . . . . . . . . . . . . . . . . . . . . .

. . . . . . . . . . . . . . . . . . . . . . . . . . . . . . . . . . . . . . . . . . . . . . . . . . . . .

Is there anything that you know of which will make the
symptoms worse?                                         Yes  /  No

If so, what? . . . . . . . . . . . . . . . . . . . . . . . . . . . . . . . . . . . . . . . . .

. . . . . . . . . . . . . . . . . . . . . . . . . . . . . . . . . . . . . . . . . . . . . . . . . . . . .

. . . . . . . . . . . . . . . . . . . . . . . . . . . . . . . . . . . . . . . . . . . . . . . . . . . . .

. . . . . . . . . . . . . . . . . . . . . . . . . . . . . . . . . . . . . . . . . . . . . . . . . . . . .

Are they worse in any particular place?                 Yes  /  No

If so, where? . . . . . . . . . . . . . . . . . . . . . . . . . . . . . . . . . . . . . . . .

. . . . . . . . . . . . . . . . . . . . . . . . . . . . . . . . . . . . . . . . . . . . . . . . . . . . .

. . . . . . . . . . . . . . . . . . . . . . . . . . . . . . . . . . . . . . . . . . . . . . . . . . . . .

. . . . . . . . . . . . . . . . . . . . . . . . . . . . . . . . . . . . . . . . . . . . . . . . . . . . .

B

Do you now

Wheeze? Yes / No

Get out of breath easily? Yes / No

Have a frequent dry cough? Yes / No

Cough at night? Yes / No

Suffer from frequent chest infections? Yes / No

Suffer from frequent ear infections? Yes / No

Have a lot of sore throats Yes / No

Have difficulty in hearing? Yes / No

Have you suffered from any severe illnesses? Yes / No

. . . . . . . . . . . . . . . . . . . . . . . . . . . . . . . . . . . . . . . . . . . .

Have you had any operations? Yes / No

Nature of operation(s) and date(s) . . . . . . . . . . . . . . . . . . . . . . . . .

. . . . . . . . . . . . . . . . . . . . . . . . . . . . . . . . . . . . . . . . . . . .

. . . . . . . . . . . . . . . . . . . . . . . . . . . . . . . . . . . . . . . . . . . .

Did you have any of the following in the past?

Asthma          Eczema          Bronchitis          Rhinitis          Glue ear

Recurrent chest infections          Hay fever          Tonsillitis

Recurrent ear infections

Does anyone in the family have allergies? Yes / No
(Asthma, eczema, hay fever, urticaria, food allergy, drug allergy etc.)

Please specify . . . . . . . . . . . . . . . . . . . . . . . . . . . . . . . . . . . . . .

. . . . . . . . . . . . . . . . . . . . . . . . . . . . . . . . . . . . . . . . . . . .

Does anyone in your family suffer from repeated infections? Yes / No

Please specify . . . . . . . . . . . . . . . . . . . . . . . . . . . . . . . . . . . . . .

. . . . . . . . . . . . . . . . . . . . . . . . . . . . . . . . . . . . . . . . . . . .

**Potential Allergens**

Please tick any of the following which are in your home:

| | | |
|---|---|---|
| Carpets | Mould | Feather/down Duvet |
| Central Heating | Trees | Wool Blankets |
| Pets | Furry Toys | Cigarette Smoke |
| Damp | Feather Pillows | |

Do you have any occupational exposure to allergens?        Yes  /  No

. . . . . . . . . . . . . . . . . . . . . . . . . . . . . . . . . . . . . . . . . .

. . . . . . . . . . . . . . . . . . . . . . . . . . . . . . . . . . . . . . . . . .

Do you have any hobbies?                                             Yes  /  No

. . . . . . . . . . . . . . . . . . . . . . . . . . . . . . . . . . . . . . . . . .

. . . . . . . . . . . . . . . . . . . . . . . . . . . . . . . . . . . . . . . . . .

**Diet**

Any food fads/fancies?                                               Yes  /  No

If so, please specify  . . . . . . . . . . . . . . . . . . . . . . . . . . . . . .

. . . . . . . . . . . . . . . . . . . . . . . . . . . . . . . . . . . . . . . . . .

Do you eat a lot of dairy products?                                 Yes  /  No

Do you eat a lot of junk food?                                      Yes  /  No

Do any foods upset you?                                             Yes  /  No

**Medication**

What treatments have you tried?  . . . . . . . . . . . . . . . . . . . . . . . .

. . . . . . . . . . . . . . . . . . . . . . . . . . . . . . . . . . . . . . . . . .

Have you ever reacted to a medicine?                                Yes  /  No

Please specify . . . . . . . . . . . . . . . . . . . . . . . . . . . . . . . . . . .

. . . . . . . . . . . . . . . . . . . . . . . . . . . . . . . . . . . . . . . . . .

Which, if any, have proved helpful?  . . . . . . . . . . . . . . . . . . . . . .

. . . . . . . . . . . . . . . . . . . . . . . . . . . . . . . . . . . . . . . . . .

C

# THE ROYAL NATIONAL THROAT, NOSE AND EAR HOSPITAL
## Middle Ear Dysfunction

FIRST VISIT

Child's Surname . . . . . . . . . . . . . . . . . . . . . . . . . . . . . . . . . . .

First Names . . . . . . . . . . . . . . . . . . . . . . . . . . . . . . . . . . . . . .

Date of Birth . . . . . . . . . . . . . . . . . . . . . . . . . . . . . . . . . . . . .

Address . . . . . . . . . . . . . . . . . . . . . . . . . . . . . . . . . . . . . . . . .

. . . . . . . . . . . . . . . . . . . . . . . . . . . . . . . . . . . . . . . . . . . . . .

. . . . . . . . . . . . . . . . . . . . . . . . . . . . . . . . . . . . . . . . . . . . . .

. . . . . . . . . . . . . . . . . . . . . . . . . . . . . . . . . . . . . . . . . . . . . .

Telephone Number . . . . . . . . . . . . . . . . . . . . . . . . . . . . . . . .

Hospital Number . . . . . . . . . . . . . . . . . . . . . . . . . . . . . . . . . .

**History of middle ear dysfunction**

When was the first problem with your child's ear(s) noted? . . . . . . . .

. . . . . . . . . . . . . . . . . . . . . . . . . . . . . . . . . . . . . . . . . . . . . .

What form did this take . . . . . . . . . . . . . . . . . . . . . . . . . . . . . .

. . . . . . . . . . . . . . . . . . . . . . . . . . . . . . . . . . . . . . . . . . . . . .

Does your child

| | |
|---|---|
| Have pain or discomfort in one or both ears? | Yes / No |
| Have a sense of fullness in one or both ears? | Yes / No |
| Suffer from frequent ear infections? | Yes / No |
| Have difficulty in hearing? | Yes / No |
| Hear ringing in the ears | Yes / No |
| Do you think your child was/is late in talking? | Yes / No |
| Do you think your child is difficult to understand? | Yes / No |

Is your child falling behind at school                 Yes / No

Is your child becoming irritable?                   Yes / No

Have a lot of sore throats?                       Yes / No

Are there any other problems or difficulties which may be relevant? . .

. . . . . . . . . . . . . . . . . . . . . . . . . . . . . . . . . . . . . . . . . . . . .

. . . . . . . . . . . . . . . . . . . . . . . . . . . . . . . . . . . . . . . . . . . . .

**Allergy History**

**Please circle any of the following which apply to your child:**

Running nose          Clear fluid discharge

                       Thick fluid discharge, often green/yellow

Catarrh going down the back of the throat

Sneezing

Blocked nose         left side         right side         both sides

Snoring

Mouth breathing at night

Itchy nose

Rubs nose with fingers/hand

Lacks sense of smell

Lacks sense of taste

Conjunctivitis

Has asthma

Wheezes

Gets out of breath easily

Has a night cough

Has a frequent dry cough

Has frequent chest infections

Has an itchy rash occasionally

Has eczema

Has headaches with vomiting

Has recurrent bouts of abdominal pain

When did these symptoms start? . . . . . . . . . . . . . . . . . . . . . . . . . .

. . . . . . . . . . . . . . . . . . . . . . . . . . . . . . . . . . . . . . . . . . . . . .

Are they worse at any particular time of year?          Yes / No

If so, when? . . . . . . . . . . . . . . . . . . . . . . . . . . . . . . . . . . . . . . .

. . . . . . . . . . . . . . . . . . . . . . . . . . . . . . . . . . . . . . . . . . . . . .

Are they worse at any particular time of day?          Yes / No

If so, when? . . . . . . . . . . . . . . . . . . . . . . . . . . . . . . . . . . . . . . .

. . . . . . . . . . . . . . . . . . . . . . . . . . . . . . . . . . . . . . . . . . . . . .

Is there anything that you know of which will make the symptoms
worse?          Yes / No

If so, what? . . . . . . . . . . . . . . . . . . . . . . . . . . . . . . . . . . . . . . .

. . . . . . . . . . . . . . . . . . . . . . . . . . . . . . . . . . . . . . . . . . . . . .

Are they worse in any particular place?          Yes / No

If so, where? . . . . . . . . . . . . . . . . . . . . . . . . . . . . . . . . . . . . . .

**Birth History**

Was the pregnancy normal?          Yes / No

If not, please specify what problems occurred . . . . . . . . . . . . . . . . . .

. . . . . . . . . . . . . . . . . . . . . . . . . . . . . . . . . . . . . . . . . . . . . .

| Labour | Normal | Rapid | Prolonged | |
|--------|--------|-------|-----------|--|
| Delivery | Normal | Forceps | Breech | Caesarian |
| Full term | | | | Yes / No |

If not, at how many weeks? . . . . . . . . . . . . . . . . . . . . . . . . . . . .

Birth weight . . . . . . . . . . . . . . . . . . . . . lb/oz

. . . . . . . . . . . . . . . . . . . . . . . . . . . . . . . kg

Condition at birth

Normal                    Difficulty with breathing             Jaundice

**Feeding**

Breastfed?                                                 Yes / No

If so, for how long? . . . . . . . . . . . . . . . . . . . . . . . . . . . . . . . .

Bottle-fed?                                             Yes / No

When was bottled milk first given? . . . . . . . . . . . . . . . . . . . . . . .

Type of milk used . . . . . . . . . . . . . . . . . . . . . . . . . . . . . . . . . . .

Did the baby feed well?                               Yes / No

If not, what problems occurred . . . . . . . . . . . . . . . . . . . . . . . . . .

. . . . . . . . . . . . . . . . . . . . . . . . . . . . . . . . . . . . . . . . . . . . . . .

. . . . . . . . . . . . . . . . . . . . . . . . . . . . . . . . . . . . . . . . . . . . . . .

Any colic?                                               Yes / No

When was weaning first started? . . . . . . . . . . . . . . . . . . . . . . . . .

Which foods were introduced? . . . . . . . . . . . . . . . . . . . . . . . . . .

. . . . . . . . . . . . . . . . . . . . . . . . . . . . . . . . . . . . . . . . . . . . . . .

Has your baby suffered from any severe illnesses?     Yes / No

Which? . . . . . . . . . . . . . . . . . . . . . . . . . . . . . . . . . . . . . . . . . . .

. . . . . . . . . . . . . . . . . . . . . . . . . . . . . . . . . . . . . . . . . . . . . . .

Has your child had any operations?                Yes / No

Nature of operation(s) and date(s) . . . . . . . . . . . . . . . . . . . . . . . .

. . . . . . . . . . . . . . . . . . . . . . . . . . . . . . . . . . . . . . . . . . . . . . .

. . . . . . . . . . . . . . . . . . . . . . . . . . . . . . . . . . . . . . . . . . . . . . .

## Family History

Are there any other children in the family?                    Yes / No

Please give the age and sex of each one ....................

.............................................................

.............................................................

Does anyone in the family have allergies?                    Yes / No
(Asthma, eczema, hay fever, urticaria, food allergy, drug allergy etc.)

Please specify .............................................

.............................................................

.............................................................

Does anyone in the family suffer from repeated infections?    Yes / No

Please specify .............................................

.............................................................

## Potential Allergens

Please tick any of the following which are in your home:

| Carpets | Mould | Feather/down Duvet |
| Central Heating | Trees | Wool Blankets |
| Pets | Furry Toys | Cigarette Smoke |
| Damp | Feather Pillows | |

## Diet

Any food fads or fancies?                                     Yes / No

If so, please specify ......................................

.............................................................

.............................................................

Does he/she eat a lot of dairy produce?                      Yes / No

Does he/she eat a lot of junk food?                          Yes / No

Do any foods upset your child?                               Yes / No

## Medications

What treatments has your child tried? . . . . . . . . . . . . . . . . . . . . . . .

. . . . . . . . . . . . . . . . . . . . . . . . . . . . . . . . . . . . . . . . . . . . . . . . . .

Has your child ever reacted to medicine?          Yes / No

Please specify . . . . . . . . . . . . . . . . . . . . . . . . . . . . . . . . . . . . . . . . .

. . . . . . . . . . . . . . . . . . . . . . . . . . . . . . . . . . . . . . . . . . . . . . . . . .

Which, if any, have proved helpful?   . . . . . . . . . . . . . . . . . . . . . . . .

# Appendix 5

## Addresses for suppliers of rhinology laboratory equipment

**Acoustic Rhinometer and Rhinomanometer**
GM Instruments Ltd.
Unit 6 Ashgrove
Ashgrove Road
Kilwinning
KA13 6PU
Scotland
Tel: +44 (0)1294 54664

**Youlten Nasal Inspiratory Peak Flow Meters**
Clement Clarke International Ltd.
Edinburgh Way, Harlow
Essex, CM20 2TT
United Kingdom
Tel: +44 (0)1279 414969
Fax: +44 (0)1279 456305
Web: http://www.clement-clarke.com

**Micro Spirometer**
Micro Med Ltd.
P.O. Box 6
Rochester
Kent
ME1 2AZ
Tel: +44 (0)1634 843383

**Smell Threshold Test**
Olfacto-Laboratories
P.O. Box 757
El Cerrito
CA 94530
U.S.A.

**Norimed (8 item smell test with pictures)**
Medizin Technik
Heimstrasse 46
CH-8953 Dietikan
Tel: +41 (0)1743 4060
Fax: +41(0)1743 4065
Email: norimed@swissonline.ch

**UPS IT Smell Identification Test**
Sensonics Inc.
P.O. Box 112
Haddon Height
NJ 08035
U.S.A.
Tel: +1 606 5477702

**Rhinoprobe**
Apotex Scientific Inc.
2100 Road to Six Flags East
Arlington
Texas 76011
U.S.A.
Tel: +1 (817) 277 0700/+1 (800) 654 0146
Fax: +1 (817) 861 8610

**House Dust Mite and Allergen Avoidance (Video)**
The Institute of Laryngology and Otology
University College London
330–332 Gray's Inn Road
London WC1X 8EE
Tel: +44 (0)20 7915 1592
Fax: +44 (0)20 7837 9279

# Appendix 6

## Normal values for peak expiratory flow rate

### A. Adults

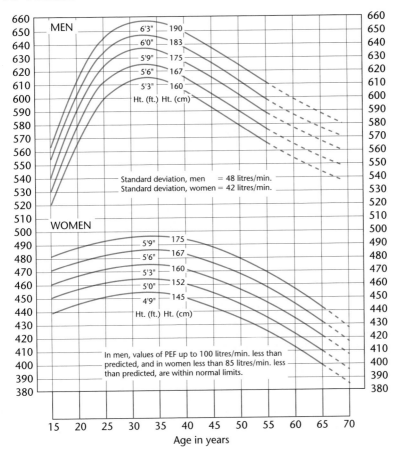

MEN

| Ht. (ft.) | Ht. (cm) |
|---|---|
| 6'3" | 190 |
| 6'0" | 183 |
| 5'9" | 175 |
| 5'6" | 167 |
| 5'3" | 160 |

WOMEN

| Ht. (ft.) | Ht. (cm) |
|---|---|
| 5'9" | 175 |
| 5'6" | 167 |
| 5'3" | 160 |
| 5'0" | 152 |
| 4'9" | 145 |

Standard deviation, men = 48 litres/min.
Standard deviation, women = 42 litres/min.

In men, values of PEF up to 100 litres/min. less than predicted, and in women less than 85 litres/min. less than predicted, are within normal limits.

Age in years

## B. Children

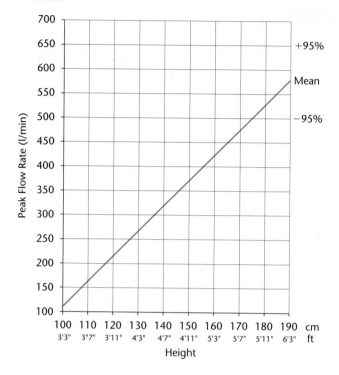

# Appendix 7

## Investigation of smell disorders

Patients with disorders of smell are often very troubled by their condition. They are also at risk from fire and dangerous gases and so should be encouraged to have smoke and gas alarms at home.

Nasal obstruction, especially nasal polyps, can cause problems with smell, which is reversible. Pateints with an intranasal foreign body may have a characteristic odour noticed by others, but not by themselves.

There are congenital conditions which cause a decrease in the ability either to detect certain smells or complete anosmia (eg) Kallmann's Syndrome, which is associated with hypogonadotrophic hypogonadism.

Patients with neurological disorders such as head injuries, temporal lobe and uncinate epilepsy and intracranial tumours can suffer olfactory disturbances.

Other possible causes include head trauma, exposure to a variety of volatile chemicals such as benzene, ethylacetate, formaldehyde, and hydrazine, paint solvents and possibly industrial dusts.

Olfactory disturbances and halluciations can occur in psychiatric states such as depression, chronic hallucinatory and confusional states and schizophrenia.

Malingerers usually deny the ability to detect substances such as ammonia or petrol, which stimulate the 5th nerve.

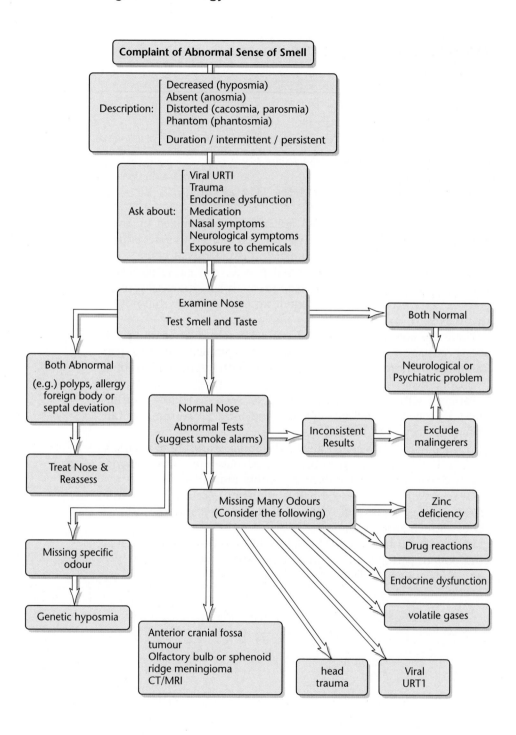

# Index